Biodynamic Excisional Skin Tension Lines for Cutaneous Surgery

Sharad P. Paul

Biodynamic Excisional Skin Tension Lines for Cutaneous Surgery

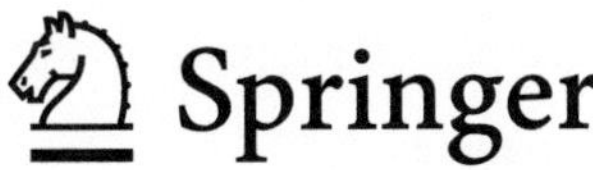 Springer

Sharad P. Paul
School of Medicine
University of Queensland
Queensland
Australia

ISBN 978-3-319-71494-3   ISBN 978-3-319-71495-0   (eBook)
https://doi.org/10.1007/978-3-319-71495-0

Library of Congress Control Number: 2018930528

Printed on acid-free paper

This Springer imprint is published by the registered company Springer International Publishing AG part of Springer Nature
The registered company address is: Gewerbestrasse 11, 6330 Cham, Switzerland

About This Book

Surgical literature is inundated with references to Langer's lines, cleavage lines, wrinkle lines and relaxed skin tension lines. The author undertook a detailed review and conducted original research to understand the 'state of the art' of skin lines in cutaneous surgery and concludes that incisional and excisional lines are different biomechanically. This book introduces the concept of biodynamic excisional skin tension (BEST) lines.

The problem with current concepts of skin tension lines is that they seem to differ in different textbooks—lines for surgical egress which work in conditions of low tension are not necessarily suitable for skin cancer surgery that has been the focus of this author's pioneering work. The book covers skin biomechanics, the properties of collagen and elastin, skin vascularity and also maps BEST lines across the body, making it a great reference guide for plastic or dermatologic surgery worldwide.

This book is an important work in the field of surgical foundations and relooks at the concept of skin lines. It is a major new work in the field of surgical research. There has been no complete treatise devoted to this topic of skin lines since Langer's original work in 1861. It will be beneficial for anyone performing cutaneous surgery and skin cancer excisions in clinical practice or for those planning further research into skin biomechanics to read this volume. It is a must-read for anyone with an interest in cutaneous surgery especially the surgeon-scientist.

Contents

Contents ix

About the Author

Sharad P. Paul initially embarked on surgical training in general/plastic surgery before establishing an integrated skin cancer practice. He has worked as a surgical consultant in public/teaching hospitals and also in primary care. Since 1996, Dr. Paul has performed over 45,000 skin cancer operations and treated over 100,000 patients—making him known for having one of the largest series of skin cancer cases anywhere in the world.

He is a senior lecturer (skin cancer) at the School of Medicine of the University of Queensland, Australia, and an honorary senior lecturer at the Department of Surgery of the University of Auckland. He is also an adjunct professor at the Auckland University of Technology. Given these academic and teaching attachments, he has a long list of conference keynote presentations and publications in peer-reviewed journals. He is a fellow of the Skin Cancer College of Australasia and was awarded the distinguished fellowship of the Royal NZ College of General Practitioners. In 2015, he was awarded the Ko Awatea International Excellence Award for leading (health) improvement on a global scale—with the citation noting 'Dr. Sharad Paul's role in improving skin cancer management, education and patient-centred care internationally, across several countries'. In 2012, he was awarded New Zealand Medical Association's highest award, the Chair's Award. In 2008, he was featured in international editions of TIME magazine in an article titled "Open Heart Surgeon"—noting his medical and humanitarian endeavours.

Introduction

Chirurgia Facit Saltum

Understanding the development of surgical methods itself becomes a fascinating philosophical pursuit. When it comes to natural science, the adage that applies is natura non facit saltum—borrowed from Carl Linnaeus by Charles Darwin for his *Origin of Species* and later adopted as a motto by Alfred Marshall for his *Principles of Economics*; it simply means 'nature does not make a leap'. In other words, changes in the natural world happen slowly and incrementally [1]. Darwin wrote: 'Multiform difficulties will occur to everyone on this theory. Most can I think be satisfactorily answered—"natura non facit saltum" answers some of the most obvious—the slowness of the change, and only a very few undergoing change at any one time answers other [2]'.

Thomas Kuhn in his seminal work, *The Structure of Scientific Revolutions* [3], sought to understand the nature of scientific innovation and concluded that when it came to breakthroughs in science, *natura non facit saltum* did not apply. Kuhn felt that dominant views of the history of science failed to capture the necessity for major scientific achievement—the abandonment of old paradigms and the introduction of new ways of thinking or applying technology. Kuhn wrote [4]: 'One cannot move from the old to the new simply by adding to what was already known [...] nor one can fully describe the new in the vocabulary used by the old and vice-versa'. Advances or new developments in surgical or medical techniques have often been stymied by existing paradigms. Kuhn coined the word 'paradigm shift' that has become so commonplace that it is part of an ironic narrative, a process where old ideas end up crushed by the audaciousness of new thinking.

Ian Hacking, the philosopher, explains further [5]: 'Normal science does not aim at novelty but at clearing up the status quo. It tends to discover what it expects to discover'. Kuhn's model can be simplified by this flow chart: Paradigm → Normal Science → Anomalies → New Paradigm.

The acceptance of a paradigm nowadays becomes the occasion for the formation of a new professional subdiscipline, with its own journals, scientific societies and textbooks. Once a paradigm is accepted, the individual scientist almost takes it for granted. He need no longer 'attempt to build his field anew, starting from first principles and justifying the use of each concept introduced' [6]. We have seen this repeatedly—the reluctance to abandon sentinel node biopsies in melanoma, well after the evidence has passed, being just one example. Strenuous and diligent attempts force 'nature' into conceptual boxes by a professional medical system that makes specialties function within silos, or behave fiscally like cartels. Set paradigms obliterate possibilities of change, and therefore, startling advances in medicine do not often happen due to practicing physicians, but often despite them.

Kuhn wasn't a philosopher, he was a physicist. Interestingly, it was his study of Aristotle that first led him towards his ground-breaking treatise on scientific revolutions. Kuhn wrote [7]: 'I approached Aristotle's texts with the Newtonian mechanics I had previously read clearly in mind. The question I hoped to answer was how much mechanics Aristotle had known, how much he had left for people like Galileo and Newton to discover. Given that formulation, I rapidly discovered that Aristotle had known almost no mechanics at all. Everything was left for his successors, mostly those of the sixteenth and seventeenth centuries. That conclusion was standard, and it might in principle have been right. But I found it bothersome because, as I was reading him, Aristotle appeared not only ignorant of mechanics, but a dreadfully bad physical scientist as well. About motion, in particular, his writings seemed to me full of egregious errors, both of logic and of observation'. Later Kuhn realized his failure to understand Aristotle was only because he was entrapped by the world of his own learned paradigms. This led him towards his theories of paradigm shifts that explain how even great scientists coexist within intellectual frameworks—and led to his conclusion that without stepping outside the frame, it is easy to miss seeing the whole picture—and in the process, Kuhn changed the way in which we view new scientific advances.

Paradigms in Skin Lines

While Langer's lines are the best-known skin lines, the observation that skin lines deformed into shapes other than that of the wounding instrument was first noted by a French surgeon, Baron Guillaume Dupuytren, when he examined a stab wound victim—noting that while the puncture wounds had been caused by an awl (a pointed round-tipped tool used to punch holes in leather), the resultant skin defects appeared longitudinal—rather like knife wounds [8]. In 1861, Langer published his treatise where he acknowledged Dupuytren's observation [9]. Langer used an awl that was 2 mm in diameter which he inserted to a depth of 2.5 cm. He marked out the resultant axes of the defects following the direction in which skin tension predominated [9]. These lines that he considered static lines of maximal tension became known as 'Langer's lines' [10]. In 1892, over 30 years after Langer's observations, Emile Kocher, a Swiss surgeon, advocated that incisions must follow Langer's lines and these became de facto surgical lines for over a century—echoing Kuhn's theory that if a paradigm becomes established, it becomes 'normal science' without much opposition.

Around 80 years after Langer, in 1941, Cox, of Manchester in England, used the same method of using a round-tipped marlinspike to map out cleavage lines of the skin. A student of the history of skin lines may have been surprised that nearly a century later Cox was still repeating the methodology of Langer's old experiments in a re-testing of the paradigm—and that the report of his results would be successfully published in major surgical journals [11]. It must be noted that Cox, however, excluded obese individuals and people with large dispositions as he felt skin tension due to their body weight would affect his measurements.

In 1963 and 1974, Alberto Bulacio Nunez of Argentina published two papers on a 'new theory' regarding the lines of skin tension [12, 13]. Except, they weren't new. Again, the methods were those used by Langer, except Bulacio used a punch biopsy instrument and also studied skin graft sites. In his second paper [13], Bulacio compared them with Cornelius Kraissl's theory of excising wounds along wrinkle lines [14]. Kraissl had felt Langer's lines, being cadaveric in origin, could not apply to the living due to the absence of muscle contractions [14]. Kraissl went on to produce composite sketches based on photographs—where patients were asked to contract facial muscles, wherein facial wrinkles were exaggerated [15].

A century after Langer, Borges attempted to change the paradigm of skin lines. He did not use a wounding instrument. Borges's method involved pinching skin and noting the direction of the ridges and furrows. He felt his method excluded false lines caused by muscle contractions and joint mobilization, and he coined the term 'relaxed skin tension lines' (RSTL) that came into routine surgical parlance [16].

In the twelfth century, John of Salisbury (Johannes Parvus, also known as 'John the Little') wrote in his book *Metalogicon*: 'Bernard of Chartres used to compare us to dwarfs perched on the shoulders of giants. He pointed out that we see more and farther than our predecessors, not because we have keener vision or greater height, but because we are lifted up and borne aloft on their gigantic stature' [17]. While the science of surgery can only advance by the introduction of new paradigms, we remain indebted to previous research and their attempts to progress the state of the art. *Nanos gigantum humeris insidentes*—in writing this treatise, I am a dwarf standing on the shoulders of giants, thereby deforming their skin lines by the sheer weight of surgical progress.

Biodynamic Excisional Skin Tension (BEST) Lines, a New Paradigm

One of the failings of previous research into skin lines was the lack of differentiation between incisional and excisional skin lines. Langer's and later Cox's experiments used small-diameter puncturing instruments and the 'cleavage lines' that resulted were noted. These studies resulted in deformation of the underlying structures of the skin in a manner expected in *incisional* surgery. While Langer conducted second experiments with larger defects, these were also in cadavers, and muscle contractions could not be accounted for.

A few years ago, I began work on a computerized tensiometer (Fig. 1), especially to study biodynamic excisional skin tension (BEST) lines [18]. More and more, I became aware that each of us has some existing pre-tension on our skin and this is often determined by body weight or body site or joint movement. That is why in certain anatomic locations of the human body, especially in areas like the lower limb, a wound that appears closeable ends up needing a skin graft. And when *excisional* wounds are created, especially greater than 8 mm, previous concepts of cleavage lines don't apply, and what matters for both cosmesis and wound healing is wound closure under least tension, and hence we must view incisional and excisional lines differently. This became a journey that led to mapping *biodynamic excisional skin tension* (BEST) lines across the body, studying skin biodynamics,

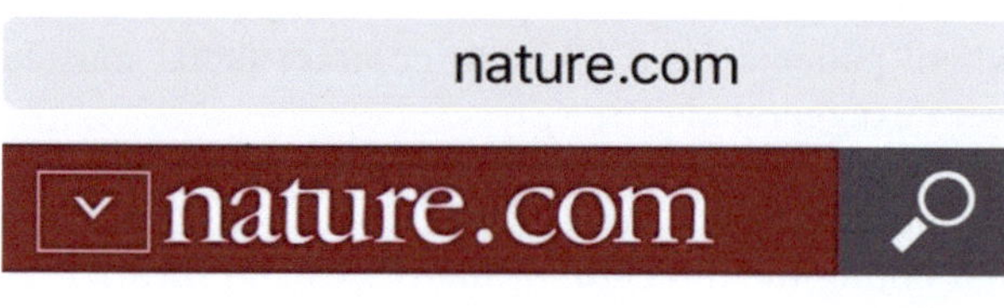

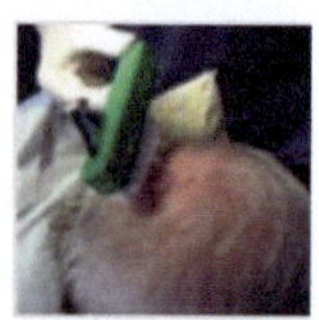

Sharad P. Paul, Justin Matulich & Nick Charlton

Scientific Reports **6**, 30117

Fig. 1 Computational analyses to understand and map biodynamic excisional skin tension lines

behaviour and cutaneous biology—a prolonged period of cutaneous introspection into the best lines for excisional surgery. I must thank people at the University of Queensland who insisted that such a study must be deserving of another research degree, and I am grateful to people who ended up as my Ph.D. supervisors—Associate Professor Cliff Rosendahl (University of Queensland) and Professor John Windsor (University of Auckland). I must especially thank Ryan Butler for many illustrations and for documenting my experiments using photography and video, Dr. Robin Hankin (Auckland University of Technology) for statistical analyses, and Natasha Paul for editorial suggestions.

The clear hazeless light of scientific research can often become an obsession, and family life is made to stand still. I must thank my family for their patience in allowing me to linger long enough on the topic to finally understand its significance.

Stephen Harper, in writing on innovation, suggests that breakthrough ideas or radical innovations usually come from outsiders. The key is to bring in people who have different perspectives [18]. Maybe having different perspectives because I work across different specialties was what led me to again revisit this already well-travelled road—and find surprising new paths. In addition to working in the field of skin cancer and being a published writer of fiction and non-fiction, I have worked in family medicine and medical law. One day a week, when I am back home, I teach creative writing to disadvantaged children—and such creativity has shown to improve science and math performance—because the creative process is nothing but a reproducible, learnable and systematic thought process [19]. Research has already demonstrated that within this structured process, revolutionary ideas can and will emerge—through a 'giant leap' and not in increments, even if this leap is only achieved through systematic thinking [19]. I hope this book offers some evidence in that regard.

Each chapter is designed to be read alone or sequentially, and therefore some basic concepts may appear recurrent. BEST lines are detailed anatomically; the face is considered last, deliberately—because BEST lines aside, there are additional surgical considerations here, such as SMAS anatomy and neurovascular zones.

Finally, I was humbled and honoured to be invited to Vienna in June 2017 (Fig. 2) to present my work in the same place where the first inquisition into skin lines was conducted by Karl Langer around 150 years ago.

Therefore, perhaps unlike nature, surgical science can progress in jumps.

Ultimately, this book is about *chirurgia facit saltum*, a leap in surgical methods that I hope will be a useful treatise for the cutaneous surgeon.

Each chapter contains research, experiments or methodology that has been peer-reviewed and published in other journals. I hope this book will help dermatological and plastic surgeons, or indeed any doctor with an interest in surgery to the skin, as much as it has advanced my own clinical work.

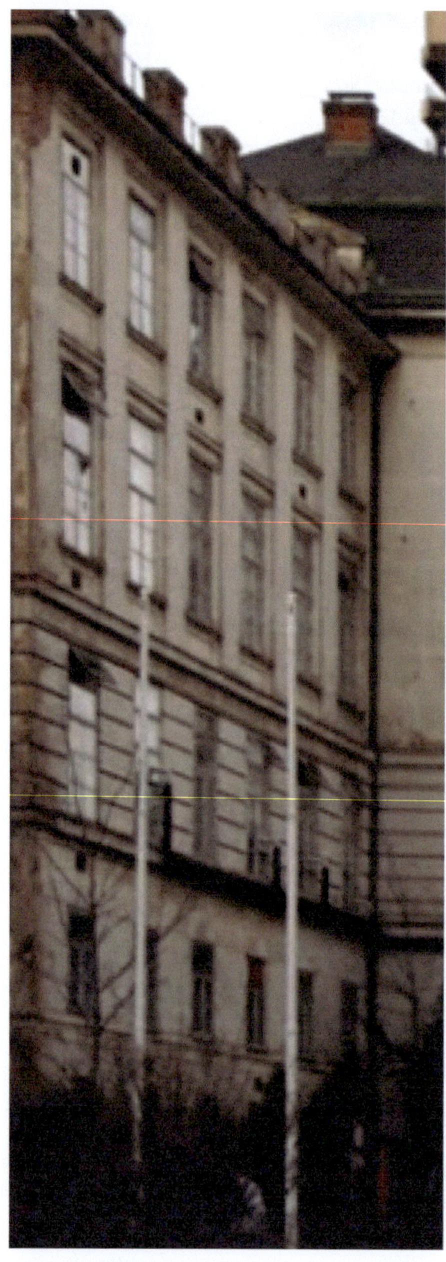

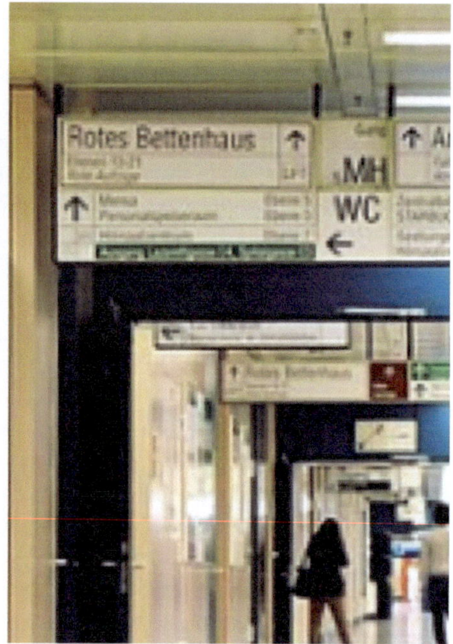

Donnerstag, 08.06.2017

è 14:00 Uhr-Seminarraum Ebene 17ç
Rotes Bettenhaus, Ebene 17.G2.04ç

Dr. Sharad Paul

"Revisiting Langer: Introducing Best
Excisional Skin Tension (BEST) Lines
of Skin"

Fig. 2 Revisiting Langer's lines: lecture introducing BEST lines, Vienna, June 2017

References

1. Fishburn G. Natura non facit saltum in Alfred Marshall (and Charles Darwin). Econ Hist Rev. 2004;40:1. https://doi.org/10.1080/18386318.2004.11681190.
2. Darwin C. The correspondence of Charles Darwin, vol. 6. Cambridge: Cambridge University Press; 1990. p. 1856–7.
3. Kuhn TS. The structure of scientific revolutions, vol. 2. Chicago: University of Chicago Press; 1970. p. 5, 16–7, 19–20, 85.
4. Kuhn TS. In: Conant J, Haugeland J, editors. The road from structure: philosophical essays 1970-1993, with an autobiographical interview. Sao Paolo: UNESP; 2006. https://doi.org/10.5007/1808-1711.2012v16n2p345.
5. Hacking I. Introduction. In: Kuhn TS, editor. The structure of scientific revolutions: 50th anniversary edition. Chicago: University of Chicago Press; 2012.
6. McWhinney IR. Changing models: the impact of Kuhn's theory on medicine. Fam Pract. 1983;1(1):3.
7. Kruger L, Lorraine JD, Heidelberger M. The probabilistic revolution, vol. I: Ideas in history. Cambridge: MIT Press; 1987. p. 7–22.
8. Dupuytren JF. Traite theorique et practique des blessure par armes de querre, vol. 1. Paris: J. B. Baillere; 1834.
9. Langer K. On the anatomy and physiology of the skin: the cleavability of the cutis (translated from Langer K. 1861. Zur Anatomie und Physiologie der Haut. II. Die Spannung der Cutis. Sitzungsbericht der mathematisch-naturwissenschaftlichen Classe der Kaiserlichen Academie der Wissenchaften, 44,19). Br J Plast Surg. 1978;3:3–8.
10. Edlich RF, Carl AB. Predicting scar formation: from ritual practice (Langer's lines) to scientific discipline (static and dynamic skin tensions). J Emerg Med. 1998;16:759–60.
11. Cox HT. The cleavage lines of the skin. Br J Surg. 1941;29:234–40. https://doi.org/10.1002/bjs.18002911408.
12. Bulacio Nunez AW, Marino H. A new procedure for investigation of tension lines of the skin. Plast Reconstr Surg. 1963;31:602.
13. Bulacio Nunez AW. A new theory regarding the lines of skin tension. Plast Reconstr Surg. 1974;53:663–9.
14. Kraissl CJ, Conway H. Excision of small tumors of the skin of the face with special reference to the wrinkle lines. Surgery. 1949;25:592.
15. Kraissl CJ. The selection of appropriate lines for elective surgical incisions. Plast Reconstr Surg. 1951;8:1–28.
16. Borges AF. Relaxed skin tension lines (RSTL) versus other skin lines. Plast Reconstr Surg. 1984;73:144–50.
17. MacGarry DD. The metalogicon of John Salisbury: a twelfth-century defense of the verbal and logical arts of the Trivium (Translated by MacGarry, Daniel Doyle). Berkeley: University of California Press; 1955. p. 167.
18. Paul SP, et al. A new skin tensiometer device: computational analyses to understand biodynamic excisional skin tension lines. Sci Rep. 2016;6:30117. https://doi.org/10.1038/srep30117.
19. Harper SC, Porter TW. Innovate or die. Ind Eng. 2011;43(9):34–9.

Chapter 1
Examining the Science Behind Skin Lines Currently Used for Surgical Excisions, and Introducing a New Concept of BEST (Biodynamic Excisional Skin Tension) Lines

1.1 History and Review of Skin Lines

The observation that clefts created in skin were shaped differently to the shape of the injury-causing instrument was noted by Baron Guillaume Dupuytren, a French anatomist and military surgeon in 1831 [1]. Dupuytren had been called to attend an attempted suicide where the patient history suggested the wounding instrument was a round-tipped stiletto. Dupuytren was in doubt as to the assertions of his patient that the wounds had been inflicted using a round-bladed stiletto because the deformities of the skin clefts suggested an instrument with a linear cutting edge. The first published anatomical account describing "cleavage lines" was that of Karl Langer, of Vienna, in 1861 [2]. Langer was to become Professor of Anatomy at Joseph's Academy in Vienna [3]. Because Langer's original paper was written in German [4], it took over a century before his work was noted by the English-speaking plastic surgical community [3]. However, in trying to make Langer's work available, Gibson still omitted a considerable portion as he found the "descriptive anatomy most boring" [3]. Langer used the term "Spaltbarkeit" which was translated into English as "cleavability" by Gibson, and this led to the term "cleavage lines."

1.2 Cleavage Lines

In 1892, Emil Kocher, a Swiss surgeon, suggested adopting Langer's lines as surgical lines and therefore some people called these Kocher's lines, based on Kocher's writings [5]. However, there were certain inconsistencies in these lines produced by Langer's technique—Malgaigne, for example, whose studies of skin texture and lines pre-dated Langer, and followed Dupuytren's original experiments—noted that these lines were sometimes different in people and also were not always conforming

© Springer International Publishing AG, part of Springer Nature 2018
S. P. Paul, *Biodynamic Excisional Skin Tension Lines for Cutaneous Surgery*,
https://doi.org/10.1007/978-3-319-71495-0_1

to the same anatomical pattern. However, Malgaigne did not make any specific recommendations as to their usefulness during surgery [6].

Pathological conditions visible on skin have shown distributions along cleavage lines—a report described lichen planus pigmentosus-inversus (LPPI), a rare variant of lichen planus, followed the pattern of cleavage lines [7]. The reasons for skin conditions or rashes occurring along cleavage lines is not known. One possible theory is the haematogenic dissemination of (pathologically) activated leukocytes along these lines [8].

The theory behind cleavage lines is that when a spike is thrust into the skin, "the skin yields immediately and a tension load radiates from the struck point" [9]. Networks of collagen assume an alignment parallel to these lines. Gibson and Kenedi concluded that when there was movement of collagen following the creation of cleavage lines, the lines of *least* extensibility are the original Langer's cleavage lines [10]. Eschricht studied the relationship between hair follicles and cleavage lines and concluded that the former mimic rivers or streams—and that there is a correspondence between hair follicles and cleavage lines [11].

One of the problems with cleavage lines being used as surgical lines is that there are variations between patients. For example, when Hutchinson studied cleavage lines of infants and adults, he found that in infants these lines were annular in the extremities, whereas in adult limbs they were generally longitudinal [12]. The question then arises—at what age does the pattern change? We already begin to doubt their suitability as surgical lines in all ages. Studies on contracture of skin grafts and cleavage lines suggested that graft contraction was less in the direction of cleavage lines, and these findings were both consistent and significant [13].

Langer observed that circular wounds always gaped in the same direction as his lines of cleavage [2]. But another question arose—was there a size that mattered— given the studies on skin grafts mentioned earlier? Kennedy and Cliff created square wounds with areas of 6.25 and 2.25 cm^2 and circular wounds with areas of 6.25 cm^2 in rabbits, rats and guinea pigs—and found that the wounds always gaped upon cleavage [14]; however, cleavage lines on pig wounds created by Gross stayed the same size [15]. To add to the confusion, Catty then created wounds of 1 cm on the forearms of men—and found they expanded to 1.3 cm on average after round-shaped clefts were created [16]. Unlike the findings on pigskin, Billingham and Medawar found that rabbit wounds always gaped, increasing in area by up to 50% [17]. Nunez, while studying the importance of elasticity on wound edge retraction, concluded that elastin fibres were the cause of tension along skin cleavage lines [18]. The disparity between some wounds gaping and some shrinking was explained by Ridge and Wright using the "lattice theory" [19]—this suggests skin has individual components that are subject to tension forces due to elasticity resulting in wound retraction. Wounds smaller than the rhomboidal unit (where rhomboidal patterns of collagen birefringence are evident) therefore shrink—due to the intact tensional forces in the individual dermal components—and larger clefts that disrupt more of the lattice structure will gape [20]. Bush and others in this study considered the "lattice" like Langer's "kernel" (isolated islands of skin that were created in his experiments) wherein Langer [21] also noted that wounds greater than a "kernel" were likely to gape not shrink—and experiments by Bush's team suggested this size may be 3–8 mm [20]. Ksander again reflected Nunez's views that asymmetrical retractions seen in circular punch wounds are due to an inherent asymmetry of elastic forces [22].

The other problem in considering cleavage lines as determined by Langer as de facto surgical lines is that they are changeable even in the same person. When Bush and others studied Langer's lines and their variability with facial expression, they found in 171 out of 175 cases, these cleavage lines were dynamic—with a rotational variability of up to 90°. They concluded that this rotation in the axis of mechanical tension could distort resultant scars if these lines were used for surgical incisions [23]. Further as Borges noted, Langer's lines were first studied in cadavers in rigor mortis so can hardly be considered lines of relaxation [24]. When a dissection of cleavage lines using Langer's original method was undertaken on the faces of Japanese cadavers, the lines seemed to have great individual variation. These authors noted "the parallel arrangement of the blood vessels and perivascular fibrous connective tissues (especially the collagen fibres) was the common histological finding obtained in all three regions" [25].

Many authors still advocate the use of Langer's cleavage lines as surgical incision lines on the face. Motegi noted that an incision placed at right angles to the direction of skin cleavage lines had a higher risk of haematoma and tension, and thereby a higher risk of hypertrophic scarring [26]. The authors explained this by pointing out when incisions were made at right angles to cleavage lines, these ended up at right angles to the collagen fibres—whereby the dermis stretches due to the straightening of the elastic fibres by 100–140% [27]. As we know, skin behaves elastically only at low-load levels. For example, on the feet, due to weight-bearing tissues, skin shows increased viscoelastic behaviour, i.e. strain becomes a function of load and time [28]. These load-bearing properties of elastin fibres decrease with age [29]. However, in the regions of the body like the toe, these factors are age-independent—and are due to the destruction of the elastin network rather than elastin itself [30, 31]. Skin may be anisotropic, but it does exhibit orthotropy i.e. a degree of symmetry with respect to two normal planes [32], which is due to the preferential orientation of collagen fibres [33].

There is no doubt that Langer, the first person to study cleavage lines in detail, was a pioneer. While skin needs to be considered three-dimensionally, Langer's experiments were essentially two-dimensional—even if a pioneering peek into the surgical anatomy of skin. Indeed, since Langer's study, 36 different lines have been described by surgeons over the years, without advancing the science much [34]! As Wilhelmi points out [34], Malgaigne found cleavage lines vary in different parts of the body [35], and as we have just discussed, they change with facial expression. Further cleavage lines have been shown to be prone to contractures when used over a joint [36]. And, as other authors have noted, many surgeons describe "Langer's lines" when they are in fact marking incisions along wrinkle lines [37]. Indeed, many textbooks and authors depict Langer's lines differently, when compared with Langer's original writings (Fig. 1.1); adding to the confusion, many denote the same lines as wrinkle lines. Let us now examine wrinkle lines in detail.

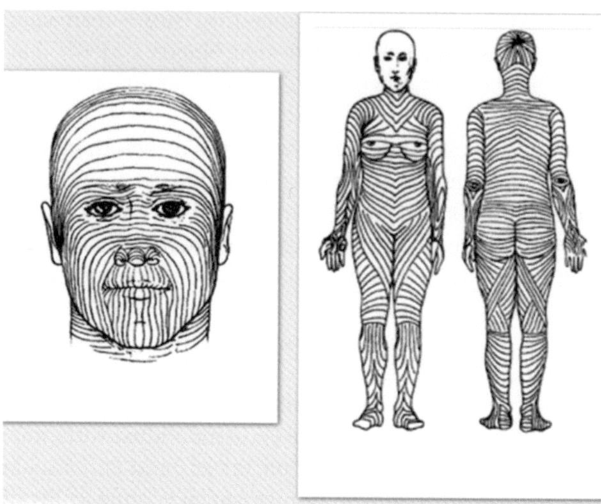

Fig. 1.1 "Skin Tension Lines of the Body Surface" portrayed here differ from Langer's original drawings—This article was published in Rosen's Emergency Medicine—Concepts and Clinical Practice 2002, Fig. 52–1 p 738; Fig. 52–2 p 739, Copyright Elsevier (2002) and reprinted with permission

1.3 Wrinkle Lines

One way of understanding wrinkles is to consider them as lines of dependency— due to gravity, and loss of suppleness of aging skin—slackness in biological membranes such as skin manifests as wrinkle lines. Wrinkle lines satisfy the one-dimensional diffusion equation that typifies the behaviour under self-weight of flexible membranes supported in a vertical plane [38]. Yet surgical practice sometimes confuses the dynamics of wrinkle lines. For example, some authors suggest pinching skin to determine wrinkle lines when they are not obvious, a method often described for relaxed skin tension that we shall discuss later in this article [39]. Tellioğlu described a technique of using a plastic adhesive sheet as a means of determining wrinkle lines [40].

As Waldorf and colleagues noted, during a discussion on planning incisions— "Many current textbooks today show and discuss wrinkle lines and RSTLs but call them Langer's lines" [41]. If experiments we discussed earlier in the article demonstrated the *dynamic* nature of Langer's lines, wrinkle lines, in contrast, are shown to be *static* lines. As Namiki and colleagues noted, "The orientations of facial static tensions were identical to the wrinkle lines in many facial areas. It is suggested that the wrinkle lines show the optimal directions of selective incisions in most facial areas except for the medial canthus and upper and lower lips" [42].

Biomechanically, Danielson considers skin a soft outer tissue of the body that behaves like an "elastic solid, consisting of a thin shell resting upon a continuum foundation" [43]. In a previous paper, his team concluded that the two main factors that affect wrinkling biomechanically are the bending stiffness of the skin and the thickness of the foundation. Bending stiffness of skin is preeminent in anatomical regions of the body where outermost tissues are extremely stiff such as the digits, and thickness of the foundation takes precedence in mobile areas such as the breasts [44]. It therefore follows that more wrinkles will be formed where the foundation is relatively thin, such as over forehead and digits—where subcutaneous tissues are very thin.

As we age, skin loses both elasticity and recoil due to the degradation of elastin fibres. UV damage or photoaging is a major causal factor of wrinkling in sun-exposed skin [45]. Wrinkles, for a cutaneous surgeon, in my view are essentially what geologists would consider fault lines—and as Griffiths noted, wrinkles that we observe on skin are essentially "marked lines that represents the bottom of the wrinkle" [46]. When skin becomes damaged due to sun-exposure one of the things that occurs is the stratum corneum becomes dryer than normal due to a lack of hyaluronic acid and this in turn creates a thicker, stiffer and fragile organ [47]. Water in sun-damaged skin ends up in a "tetrahedron form"—essentially free, and leading to a decrease in dermal compartment volume and a reduction in the subcutaneous fat compartment of skin [48], which is another occurrence that leads to wrinkling.

One of the problems in this author's view, of using wrinkle lines as surgical lines for excisional surgery (as opposed to merely placing incisions) is that there has been no demonstrable anatomical or histological basis that would suggest that these lines handle skin tension or load better. Many authors have studied this and concluded that there is no difference between wrinkles and the adjacent skin when observed histologically [49]. Piérard felt that perhaps the anatomical basis for a wrinkle under the microscope lay beneath skin in the hypodermis where trabeculae of the retinacula cutis are broader in wrinkled areas [50]. Other teams commenting on the relationship between the dermis and wrinkles—teams led by Contet-Audonneau [51] and Tsuji [52] noted a decrease in actinic damage at the bottom of the wrinkle compared to its sides or adjacent skin. Some reports have noted wrinkles may indeed be different at their depths compared to the walls of a wrinkle—Scott and Green noted chondroitin sulfate GAGs (glycosaminoglycans) are reduced under wrinkles with asymmetrical variations between its flanks probably due to differences in solar ray exposure [53]. Herein lies one of the problems in using wrinkles for elliptical excisions after skin cancer—on the wrinkle sidewalls, collagen fibres run parallel to the fold, whereas at the bottom, they are mostly perpendicular to the wrinkle [54]. To complicate matters, when operating on sun-damaged skin, which is the predominant patient group when it comes to skin cancer—studies in mice have shown that collagen is mostly in a vertical tail to head, with an orientation that corresponds to the meridian line of the body. However, in actinic damaged or UV-damaged skin, fibroblasts tend to align horizontally and synthesize horizontal collagen fibres, contradicting previous theories [55]. Others suggest that a decrease in dermal area, as compared to epidermis area, is one of the pre-requisites for the formation of a wrinkle [51]. Force loads also matter—because a loss of intra-dermal tensional strength has been noted to be a major component in the biomechanics of wrinkle formation [56].

The current surgical understanding regarding wrinkles are, in my view, almost using geological principles that are observed during the process of buckling [57]. Buckling involves two components—namely Young's modulus and thickness, and therefore one can use computational methods to calculate the likelihood of this phenomenon [58]. Kuwazuru extended this concept of buckling onto a 5-layered skin model and proposed an explanation as to why wrinkling only becomes apparent in old age [59]. The mechanical approach to wrinkling has besotted not just surgical researchers, but also biomechanical engineers. Magnenat-Thalmann studied skin wrinkling with a three-layer model and showed a gradual enlargement of the buckling-length with aging [60]. The proponents of the buckling theory of wrinkling with age explain it by suggesting that a wrinkle is initiated by the repetition of buckling caused by a muscle contraction at the same site [59]. The three-layer model was shown to simulate wrinkling better than models involving fewer layers [61]. One way of improving these multi-layer analyses is to simulate the effects of aging i.e. loss of moisture and thickness within these layers—for example there is an increase in collagen cross-links with age which makes the dermis stiffer [62]. Many computational methods are purely geometrical [63] and have not replicated wrinkling and furrowing accurately enough to help surgical science [64].

The modelling of wrinkling purely as a "fault line" or a "buckle" does not explain certain findings that indicate other biological factors at play. In animals like pigs, with age and fat deposition skin tension lines begin to run transversely, whereas in thinner animals, skin tension lines run more obliquely [65]. Wrinkles can also simply disappear, as noted in a case of a baby with Michelin Tyre Syndrome [66]. Furthering the research into wrinkling as a biological (rather than mechanical) phenomenon, researchers found that increased wrinkling may be a sign of impending heart disease, metabolic disorders, osteoporosis or degenerative disorders [67]. Tybjærg-Hansen and others studied over 10,000 Danes and found that wrinkles—especially ear lobe creases indicated the body's biological age and was an indicator for heart disease [68]. Studies on Shar Pei dogs show that wrinkling can be caused by mucinosis—high hyaluronic acid levels in both cutaneous tissues and the blood stream, and such high levels are due to an excess in the activity (overexpression) of the HAS2 enzyme [69] which can, rather paradoxically, cause wrinkling.

Mechanical approaches also do not explain accurately Borges' finding that when one pinches oneself, wrinkles become larger when they form parallel to Langer's lines [70]. Kraissl espoused a viewpoint that when cleavage lines such as Langer's lines and wrinkle lines were compared, it was the latter that were best used for surgical incisions [71]. In support of Kraissl's theory, many other authors also concluded "wrinkle lines and RSTLs largely coincide and should be used instead of Langer's lines for planning incisions" [41]. When studies were done on undermining of skin, it was shown to not affect the configuration of skin when it came to skin lines [42]. Others felt wrinkle lines were best for surgery because where wrinkle lines ran parallel to muscles, muscle contractions did not affect tension within a wrinkle [72]. And then Borges, who was widely published on the topic of skin lines, had major reservations about wrinkle lines as guides for surgical incisions when he said "relaxed skin tension lines (RSTL) are the direction of constant tension in the skin while in repose, and do not always coincide with the wrinkle lines" [73].

1.4 Relaxed Skin Tension Lines (RSTL)

After Cox [74] and Bulacio [18] replicated Langer's study, albeit with slightly different results, Rubin attempted to understand the relaxed tension lines of the face. Rubin presented a paper on skin tension lines, describing his method—making an imprint of facial skin lines using a chemical-coated paper [75].

Borges first defined the concept of relaxed skin tension lines (RSTL) [73]. When the skin is relaxed, furrows are formed—these are made more noticeable by pinching skin and noting the direction of furrows and ridges [76]. Of course these are not to be confused with sleep lines, skin lines formed due to posture or pillow pressure after relaxation [77]. A decade after he first described RSTL, Borges refined the technique of determining these lines by stating it is important to note when pinching skin one needs to consider *both* furrows and ridges—because when contour lines are produced by muscle or joint action, one only notes furrows [24].

It is also important to note that while RSTL lines were non-contentious on the face—when asked about RSTL on the rest of the body, Borges deferred to Kraissl [78], who essentially described wrinkle lines, or Courtiss's [37] technique of using Ω-shaped skin incision—both suggesting the RSTL concept on the rest of the body is essentially following wrinkle lines. Given we know wrinkle lines have no increased ability to handle load, this theory or RSTL therefore becomes biomechanically unproven—especially when one considers areas like the scalp and lower limb—both situations the author will be discussing in more detail. In many books, Langer's lines and RSTL are marked identically especially on the limbs creating confusion. In attempts to solve this conundrum, researchers studied the microanatomy [79] to determine skin tension lines—and concluded that skin tension lines are formed by the interrelation between elastin and collagen fibres, as well as fixed attachments between collagen fibres—even if Langer believed there was no elastin in his skin lines during his investigations, especially in his third article [80]. Many surgeons believe that knowledge of RSTL on the face must be a pre-requisite for, and form a fundamental part of plastic surgical training [81].

At a basic level, resting skin tension lines matter because there exists a positive correlation between tension and increased scar tissue formation [82, 83]. And, release of tension in a fibroblast populated collagen lattice results in cellular apoptosis [84]. Part of the problem is, most studies have been done after creating clefts or incisions and not after excisional surgery such as after skin cancer. The author's hypothesis that excisional lines must be biodynamically relevant, and differ based on bodily site and dimension is supported by the fact that the primary factors for relieving tension at skin edges—sutures—need to retain their tensile strength for 6 weeks to 6 months to be effective in preventing scar widening or hypertrophy [85]. Neither Langer, Borges or any other investigator sought to study the effect after *excisional* surgery and this is the reason why this author's surgical research has focused on *best excisional skin tension* (BEST) lines. In certain conditions—such as Ehlers-Danlos syndrome type I [86] and cutis laxa [87], resting skin tension lines are almost absent. Therefore, whether lines of skin tension have an anatomical basis was still a subject of scientific debate [79], and had previously never been studied properly for excisional surgery.

Kenedi and others hoped to prepare "tension maps" of the human skin surface that would indicate the magnitude and orientation of local skin tensions—but this was not accomplished because the variations were too great with their testing apparatus [88]. One way to consider skin is to consider it as a 3-D network of lines with multidirectional tensions of elastic fibres and collagen beams—and this has also contributed to the confusion between tension lines, wrinkle lines and cleavage lines [89]. As discussed earlier, skin resistance to traction predominates along Langer's lines and varies with body site. In many situations, skin tension is greater along Langer's lines [89], and their dynamic nature may accentuate their unsuitability for excisional surgery. However, in some situations like the lower limb, the situation is different when compared to facial skin. On the lower limbs Langer's lines are aligned along elastin fibres—in a study 76% were in the direction of Langer lines, and 5.1% perpendicular [89]. Skin is anisotropic i.e. has different values of tension when measured in different directions, and due to Young's modulus, the distribution angle is maximal along Langer's lines [90].

Stark developed a special compass-like instrument (each measurement only took 1.5 s)—and noted that direction of the maximum tension can be found by stretching the skin using his device with equal force—and this direction of minimum elongation is aligned along Langer's lines [91]. Borges's method, widely used in surgery is possibly the least accurate, especially in areas like the scalp or pretibial areas overlying bone. This is because other than the face, Borges's lines follow Langer's lines, and in directions against Langer's lines, they are impeded by the skin tension that ends up making them irregular [70]. Barbenel used a suction method to understand skin tension—his theory suggests that when the contour of a chamber is drawn in during suction and when this chamber is removed—an oval outline is observed instead of a circle, and its main axis corresponds to Langer's lines [92]. Zahouani experimented with using 3-D imaging—three-dimensional imaging of skin using a "signature" printed on the surface of the stratum corneum [93, 94]. It is clear from all these different methods achieving different results that skin morphology contains a network of lines whose organization reflects the multi-directional nature of elastic and collagen fibres in the superficial dermis [94] and therefore all these lines can be suitable for making incisions, but when it comes to excisional surgery especially for larger wounds, these may not be accurate.

Hashimoto [95] classified skin morphological lines by mapping this ultrastructure: with a precise four-level classification:

  (I) The primary lines are clearly marked and are between 20 and 100 µm deep
  (II) The secondary lines are more discrete and correspond to a depth of 5–40 µm and are perpendicular to the primary lines
  (III) The tertiary lines correspond to the corneocyte border (about 0.5 µm)
  (IV) The quaternary lines correspond to the morphology of each corneocyte (about 0.05 µm)

Hashimoto also concluded that lines of type (I) are ones that are visible on pinching; lines of types (III) and (IV) are not visible without microscopy [95]. Analysis of skin tension lines of Caucasian women aged between 20 and 80 years shows a decrease of the density of lines of depth <60 µm and an augmentation of deep lines beyond 60 µm—the former is due to elastin, and the latter is what we note as cleavage or tension lines [89].

One of the main reasons why incisional and excisional lines must be considered differently is because of the properties of skin extension under load—to begin with there is a rapid increase in length for very small increments of force; towards the end, relatively small extensions result from relatively large increases in force [96]. Morgan noted the final part of this curve is almost identical to the force obtained when testing pure collagen [97]. Studies have also shown that when skin is stretched and thickness of skin is measured, there comes a time when the volume decreases [98]. This is especially why in thin actinic damaged skin of the lower limb, excisional lines end up different to RSTL or wrinkle lines—resulting in skin grafts when pinching skin indicates primary closure would have been possible.

When it comes to excisional lines, the most important parameters are closing tension and extensibility i.e. how far the margins can be advanced [22], and these three forces—midline modulus, closing tension and terminal modulus [22]—can be calculated using the modulus of elasticity [99]. Some authors propose the parallel arrangement of collagen and elastic fibres is to allow collagen fibres to buckle and allow for extension of elastic fibres at low strains [100]. At high strains, the collagen fibres bear the load by straightening [100]. We also know that when it comes to excisional surgery, mechanical response of the skin can be highly asymmetric—and becomes a function of the locus and direction of the applied force vector [29]. Because the SMAS (superficial musculoaponeurotic system) layer on the face places certain parts of the face under constant tension, this asymmetry is amplified [101] and that is why RSTL lines end up ideal on the face—however this isn't the case for elsewhere. The other issue on the face is that there is improvement due to skin moisture—studies show that tension dissipation is increased by 28% after 1 month of moisturizer use [102]. To summarise the relationship between collagen and elastin, given the role of the latter in cleavage lines has been discussed—collagen fibres exist as a biaxial orientated wavy fibre network in skin [103]. Elastin makes up 2–4% of the dermis and is entwined with collagen in varying thickness and density [104]. Internal forces are transmitted from the muscles through the dermis to the epidermis and generate skin deformation that we note as skin tension lines.

1.5   Special Situations: Scalp and Lower Limb

What determines scar-formation is what happens at the dermis layer of skin—in fact, 75% of the dry weight of the dermis is due to collagen [105]—and in the scalp this is important due to the galea (aponeurosis) layer attached to the dermis. Given the occipitofrontalis muscle on the scalp, skin lines we have discussed behave differently on the scalp when compared to other areas—for example, Kraissl's [78] lines run transversely (coronal), whereas Langer's lines run vertically (sagittal) and while Borges' lines are in the same direction as Kraissl's lines, they are not identical [106]. If we decide to measure wound tension across the scalp, essentially there are two methods—Harvey's technique [107] is one of determining intraluminal pressure to disrupt a wound, while Howe's method [108] is measuring forces requited to pull apart a wound. However, in both these techniques, there has been a difficulty in the experimental method used being convenient and consistent. Previous authors have also commented on the lack of information about the forces needed to close a wound after excisional surgery [109].

The scalp is also unique because of the presence of hair follicles and the relation to skin lines. Many authors have commented on the relationship between Langer's lines and hair follicles—experimental studies have shown there is a good correlation between Langer's lines and direction of hair streams [110].

When it comes to surgical planes, we remember from our medical school days that layers of the scalp are easily remembered by the mnemonic SCALP: S (skin), C (connective tissue), A (aponeurosis), L (loose areolar tissue), and P (pericranium) [111]—skin can be easily freed up during cutaneous surgery once one is working in the loose areolar tissue plane. Stress relaxation and creep are two viscoelastic properties that aid scalp wound closure—stress relaxation is defined as the decrease in the amount of force necessary to maintain a fixed amount of skin stretch over time; creep is the gain in skin surface area that results when a constant load is applied [112]. Both these also make the scalp especially suited to the use of saline expanders, sometimes for several weeks or months [113] or even rapid intraoperative expansion [114]. Camirand and Doucet reported their comparison between parallel and perpendicular hairline incisions, and concluded that incisions perpendicular to the direction of the hair follicle allowed hair to grow through the hairline incision and end up with a more natural cosmetic appearance [115]. More than anywhere else, rotational skin flaps are employed on the scalp to close larger defects and single, double and triple flaps have been described in detail [116]. Tension is especially important on the scalp because when perfusion pressure drops below a critical closing pressure of arterioles in the sub-dermal plexus, nutritional blood flow ceases and flap ischemia occurs [117].

We know that if stress–relaxation is repeatedly applied over time deformation of the skin will result in permanent elongation [118]. The scalp tissue's stress response to displacement is tri-phasic [119]—initially linear (load range: 0–500 g), the scalp's compliance gradually reduces (load range: 500–1500 g) and eventually shows an exponential stress-strain characteristic of rapidly increasing stiffness (load range: 1500–5000 g).

However there have been very little biomechanical tension studies on scalp skin lines to understand the concepts of cleavage, tension and wrinkle lines we have been discussing, and hence this author developed a bi-directional, real-time tensiometer [120] with the specific purpose of determining biodynamic excisional skin tension (BEST) Lines for cutaneous surgery—and it wasn't a coincidence that this device was first tested on the scalp [120].

The skin tension problem is further complicated by poor vascularity, especially in older, actinic damaged patients [121]. To overcome this problem, many authors have planned island flaps on the lower limb that incorporate fasciocutaneous tissue [122]—but these often need identification of perforators using a Doppler probe [123], or are confined to specific pre-determined anatomical locations as in the case of the keystone design island perforator flap [124]. In all non-islanded flaps where the subdermal plexus is retained, there is a suppressive effect on vascular dynamics [125]. After all, one of the reasons for island flaps in the first place is to try and improve cutaneous vascularity. Notably after experimental studies on island flaps, Milton concluded, "an island is safer than a peninsula"—because when a flap is "islanded" it tends to almost solely depend on the vena comitantes rather than its arterial circulation [126]. However, the problem with these island flaps is that they may offer solutions regarding vascularity, but when it comes to wound tension or handling load, they are inadequate—especially when larger skin lesions have been removed. Random cutaneous flaps have fared poorly on the lower limb and probably because most flaps have been raised superficial to the deep fascia [127]. Haertsch conducted a dye-injection study on 22 post-mortem legs and demonstrated the role of the fascial plexus—his studies showed skin flaps in the leg can only perform reliably if the deep fascia of the leg is included—and Haertsch confirmed that for practical purposes, the "surgical plane" of the leg lies deep to the deep fascia [128].

In making a statement "the keystone flap: not an advance, just a stretch" [129], Douglas's team suggested the complete relaxation of skin in one axis (from *in vivo* length) does produce modest tension benefits in the orthogonal axis. However, the amount of increased orthogonal stretch was of the order of 1 mm, "a very minimal and dubious benefit" [130] suggesting that such island flaps do not lower wound tension significantly.

1.6 Conclusion

Elliptical incisions or cutouts while excising skin cancers are the norm—and adequate attention to skin tension that may result after excision is paramount for complication-free surgery. Therefore, proper planning is very important while planning incisions and closure [131]. Given, as we've discussed differences (and similarities) exist between Langer's cleavage lines, wrinkle lines and relaxed skin tension lines (RSTL)—and an improperly oriented excision may mean the difference between primary closure or a skin graft [132]. While undermining the wound reduces tension [133], incorrectly placed scars often result in unsightly cosmetic outcomes. The conclusion we can draw is that wrinkle lines, RSTL and Langer's lines are (and have been considered) acceptable for surgical incisions and have been employed by many surgeons. However, due to greater wound tension after *excisional* surgery, the dynamics change and these situations have not received the same surgical scientific attention.

If all these skin lines have not caused enough surgical confusion, then we can add maximal skin tension lines (MSTLs) to this mix. Leshin discusses these as "lines of surgical excision" and suggests methods of determining MSTL [134] thus: "The simplest approach is to pinch the skin in all directions to determine where the tension on the skin is least. Maximal wrinkling occurs with pinching in the direction of the short axis of the planned excision. Alternatively, having the patient move the underlying muscles by grimacing or smiling may unmask these lines" [134]. Is this not the same technique to determine RSTL? Or are wrinkle lines now being advocated as excisional lines instead of RSTL? Leshin's MSTL have been described as not always congruent to RSTL [135] or conforming to wrinkle lines [78] or to the action of underlying muscles [78]. Pinkus described "folding lines" [136] that he thought would serve for planning excisions but they are also confusing and too many to recall easily. Kraissl's lines can be considered anti-muscular lines [78] and therefore only useful for incisions (for surgical egress) or excisions (of small defects) where the load is low [71]. Striae distensae, a reflection of cellular, fibrillar, hormonal, and mechanical alterations—lines that are implicated in various pathological and physiological conditions—have also been described by authors as a possible alternative while planning surgery [137].

Another problem with all these lines when considered individually is that they seem to differ in different textbooks, and people have not separated incisional and excisional lines while studying them—lines for surgical egress which work in conditions of low tension, are not necessarily suitable for excisional surgery [138]—and as the author has noted in other articles, current practice often lacks "science" [138]—that's why this author has now introduced the term *Biodynamic Excisional Skin Tension* (BEST) Lines [138]. This book is essentially a treatise on BEST lines for cutaneous surgery.

References

1. Dupuytren G. Traité théorique et pratique des blessures par armes de guerre. Paris; 1834.
2. Langer K. On the anatomy and physiology of the skin, I: the cleavability of the cutis. Br J Plast Surg. 1978;31(1):3–8.
3. Gibson T. Karl Langer (1819–1887) and his lines. Br J Plast Surg. 1978;31(1):1–2.

 4. Langer K. Zur Anatomie und Physiologie der Haut. Über die Spaltbarkeit der Cutis. Sitzungsbericht der Mathematisch-naturwissenschaftlichen Classe der Wiener Kaiserlichen Academie der Wissenschaften 1861, Abt 44.
 5. Kocher ET. Chirurgische Operationslehre. Jena; 1982.
 6. Malgaigne JF. Traite d'anatomie Chirurgicale et de Chirurgie Experimentale. Paris: J.B. Baillie're; 1834.
 7. Peng W, Tan C. Lichen planus pigmentosus-inversus following Langer's lines of cleavage: a rare clinical presentation. Dermatol Sin. 2015;33:241–2.
 8. Wollenberg A, Eames T. Skin diseases following a Christmas tree pattern. Clin Dermatol. 2011;29:189–94.
 9. Faga A. A new method to visualize Langer's lines. J Dermatol Surg Oncol. 1981;7(1):53–5.
10. Gibson T, Kenedi RM. The structural components of the dermis and their mechanical characteristics. In: Montagna W, Bentley JP, Dobson RL, editors. Advances in biology of skin, vol. 10. New York: Appleton-Century-Crofts; 1970. p. 34–7.
11. Eschricht K. Ueber die Richtung der Haare am menschlichen Koerpen, Miiller's Arch. 1837, rec. by Poirot P and Charpy A. Traite d'Anatomie Hurnaine. Paris: Masson; 1899. p. 886.
12. Hutchinson C, Koop CE. Lines of cleavage in the skin of the newborn infant. Anat Rec. 1956;126:299–310.
13. Sawhney CP, Monga HL. Wound contraction in rabbits and the effectiveness of skin grafts in preventing it. Br J Plast Surg. 1971;24(3):233–7.
14. Kennedy DF, Cliff WJ. A systemic study of wound contraction in mammalian skin. J Pathol. 1979;11:207–22.
15. Gross JP, Farinelli W, Sadow P, Anderson R, Bruns R. On the mechanism of skin wound "contraction": a granulation tissue "knockout" with a normal phenotype. Proc Natl Acad Sci U S A. 1995;12:5982–6.
16. Catty RHC. Healing and contraction of experimental full thickness wounds in the human. Br J Surg. 1965;52:542–8.
17. Billingham RE, Medawar PB. Contracture and intussusceptive growth in the healing of extensive wounds in mammalian skin. J Anat. 1955;89:114–23.
18. Bulacio Nuñez AW. A new theory regarding the lines of skin tension. Plast Reconstr Surg. 1974;53:663–9.
19. Ridge MD, Wright V. The directional effects of skin. A bioengineering study of skin, with particular reference to Langer's lines. J Invest Dermatol. 1966;46:341–34.
20. Bush JA, Ferguson MWJ, Mason T, McGrouther DA. Skin tension or skin compression? Small circular wounds are likely to shrink, not gape. J Plast Reconstr Aesthet Surg. 2008;61(5):529–34.
21. Langer K. On the anatomy and physiology of the skin II. Skin tension. Br J Plast Surg. 1978;31:93–106.
22. Ksander GA, Vistnes LM, Rose EH. Excisional wound biomechanics, skin tension lines and elastic contraction. Plast Reconstr Surg. 1977;59(3):398–406.
23. Bush J, Ferguson MW, Mason T, McGrouther G. The dynamic rotation of Langer's lines on facial expression. J Plast Reconstr Aesthet Surg. 2007;60:393–9.
24. Borges AF. Relaxed skin tension lines (RSTL) versus other skin lines. Plast Reconstr Surg. 1984;73:144–50.
25. Nakano Y, Motegi K. Orientation of cleavage lines, fibrous connective tissues and blood vessels in the facial skin. J Maxillofac Surg. 1983;11(2):58–63.
26. Motegi K. Consideration of the formation and biological significance of hypertrophic scar. J Maxillofac Surg. 1984;12:123–7.
27. Niijima Y. The structure of connective tissues. J Japan Med Soc. 1962;4:374.
28. Reihsner R, Balogh B, Menzel EJ. Two-dimensional elastic properties of human skin in terms of an incremental model at the in vivo configuration. Med Eng Phys. 1995;17(4):304–13.
29. Daly CH, Odland GF. Age-related changes in the mechanical properties of human skin. J Invest Dermatol. 1979;73:84–7.

30. Escoffier C, de Rigal J, Rochefort A, Vasselet R, Leveque JL, Agache PG. Age-related mechanical properties of human skin: an in vivo study. J Invest Dermatol. 1989;93(3):353–7.
31. Lanir Y. A structural theory for the homogeneous biaxial stress-strain relationship in flat collagenous tissue. J Biomech. 1979;12:423–36.
32. Lanir Y, Fung YC. Two-dimensional mechanical properties of rabbit skin. I. Experimental system. J Biomech. 1974;7(1):29–34.
33. Lanir Y, Fung YC. Two-dimensional mechanical properties of rabbit skin. II. Experimental results. J Biomech. 1974;7(2):171–82.
34. Wilhelmi BJ, Blackwell SJ, Phillips LG. Langer's lines: to use or not to use. Plast Reconstr Surg. 1999;104(1):208–14.
35. Malgaigne JF. Traité d'anatomie chirurgicale et de chirurgie expérimentale. Paris: J.B. Baillie're; 1838.
36. Blocker TG, Hendrix JH, Herrmann GC, Hall E. Application of technics of reconstructive surgery to certain problems in general surgery. Ann Surg. 1949;129(6):777–82.
37. Courtiss EH, Longarcre JJ, deStefano GA, et al. The placement of elective skin incisions. Plast Reconstr Surg. 1963;31:31–44.
38. Mansfield EW. Gravity-induced wrinkle lines in vertical membranes. Proc R Soc Lond. 1981;375:307–25.
39. Jankauskas S, Cohen IK, Grabb WC. Basic techniques of plastic surgery. In: Smith JW, Aston SJ, editors. Plastic surgery. 4th ed. Boston: Little, Brown and Company; 1991.
40. Tellioğlu AT. Determination of wrinkle lines with a transparent adhesive sheet. Plast Reconstr Surg. 2001;108(3):803–4.
41. Waldorf JC, Perdikis G, Terkonda SP. Planning incisions. Oper Tech Gen Surg. 2002;4(3):199–206.
42. Namiki Y, Fukuta K, Alani H. The directions of static skin tensions in the face: their roles in facial incisions. Ann Plast Surg. 1992;28(2):147–51.
43. Danielson DA. Wrinkling of the human skin. J Biomech. 1977;10(3):201–4.
44. Danielson DA, Natarajan S. Tension field theory and the stress in stretched skin. J Biomech. 1975;8:135–42.
45. Griffiths CE. The clinical identification and quantification of photodamage. Br J Dermatol. 1992;127:37–42.
46. Gilchrest BA. Skin aging and photoaging: an overview. J Am Acad Dermatol. 1989;21:610–3.
47. Tagami H. Functional characteristics of the stratum corneum in photoaged skin in comparison with those found in intrinsic aging. Arch Dermatol Res. 2008;300:S1–6.
48. Waller JM, Maibach HI. A quantitative approach to age and skin structure and function: protein, glycosaminoglycan, water, and lipid content and structure. In: Barel AO, Paye M, Maibach HI, editors. Handbook of cosmetic science and technology. 3rd ed. London: Informa Health Care; 2009. p. 243–60.
49. Bosset S, Barre P, Chalon A, Kurfurst R, Bonte F, Andre P, Nicolas J. Skin ageing: clinical and histopathologic study of permanent and reducible wrinkles. Eur J Dermatol. 2002;12:247–52.
50. Piérard GE, Lapière CM. The microanatomical basis of facial frown lines. Arch Dermatol. 1989;125:1090–2.
51. Contet-Audonneau JL, Jeanmaire C, Pauly G. A histological study of human wrinkle structures: comparison between sun-exposed areas of the face, with or without wrinkles, and sun-protected areas. Br J Dermatol. 1999;140:1038–47.
52. Tsuji T, Yorifuji T, Hayashi Y, Hamada T. Light and scanning electron microscopic studies on wrinkles in aged persons' skin. Br J Dermatol. 1986;114:329–35.
53. Scott I, Green MR. The human periorbital wrinkle. In: Baran R, Maibach HI, editors. Textbook of cosmetic dermatology. New York: Taylor & Francis; 2004. p. 277–82.
54. Humbert P, Viennet C, Legagneux K, Grandmottet F, Robin S, Oddos T, Muret P. In the shadow of the wrinkle: theories. J Cosmet Dermatol. 2012;11(1):72–8.
55. Yasui T, Takahashi Y, Ito M, Fukushima S, Araki T. Observation of dermal collagen fiber in wrinkled skin using polarization-resolved second-harmonic-generation microscopy. Opt Express. 2009;17:912–23.

56. Piérard GE, Uhoda I, Piérard-Franchimont C. From skin microrelief to wrinkles: an area ripe for investigation. J Cosmet Dermatol. 2003;2:21–8.
57. Genzer J, Groenewold J. Soft matter with hard skin: from skin wrinkles to templating and material characterization. Soft Matter. 2006;2:310–23.
58. Agache PG, Humbert P. Measuring the skin. Berlin: Springer; 2004. p. 727–57.
59. Kuwazuru O, Saothong J, Yoshikawa N. Mechanical approach to aging and wrinkling of human facial skin based on the multistage buckling theory. Med Eng Phys. 2008;30:516–22.
60. Magnenat-Thalmann N, Kalra P, Lévêque JL, Bazin R, Batisse D, Querleux B. A computational skin model: fold and wrinkle formation. IEEE Trans Inf Technol Biomed. 2002;6:317–23.
61. Flynn C, McCormack BAO. Finite element modelling of forearm skin wrinkling. Skin Res Technol. 2008;14:261–9.
62. Wulf HC, Sandby-Møller J, Kobayasi T, Gniadecki R. Skin aging and natural photoprotection. Micron. 2004;35:185–91.
63. Sang PI, Hodgins JK. Capturing and animating skin deformation in human motion. ACM Trans Graph. 2006;25:881–9.
64. Terzopoulos D, Waters K. Physically-based facial modeling, analysis, and animation. J Visual Comp Animat. 1990;1:73–80.
65. Rose EH, Vistnes LM, Ksander VA. Skin tension lines in the domestic pig. Plast Reconstr Surg. 1976;57(6):729–32.
66. Nomura Y, Ota M, Tochimaru H. Self-healing congenital generalized skin creases: Michelin tire baby syndrome. J Am Acad Dermatol 2010;63(6):1110–1.
67. Makrantonaki E, Bekou V, Zouboulis CC. Genetics and skin aging. Dermatoendocrinology. 2012;4(3):280–4.
68. Christoffersen M, Frikke-Schmidt R, Schnohr P, Jensen GB, Nordestgaard BG, Tybjærg-Hansen A. Visible age-related signs and risk of ischemic heart disease in the general population: a prospective cohort study. Circulation. 2014;129(9):990–8.
69. Universitat Autònoma de Barcelona. Why Shar Pei dogs have so many wrinkles. Science Daily. 2008; 16 Nov 2008.
70. Borges AF. Relaxed skin tension lines. Dermatol Clin. 1989;7:169–77.
71. Kraissl CJ, Conway H. Excision of small tumors of the skin of the face with special reference to the wrinkle lines. Surgery. 1949;25(4):592–600.
72. Thacker JG, Stalnecker MC, Allaire PE, Edgerton MT, Rodeheaver GT, Edlich RF. Practical applications of skin biomechanics. Clin Plast Surg. 1977;4(2):167–71.
73. Borges AF, Alexander JE. Relaxed skin tension lines, z-plasties on scars, and fusiform excision of lesions. Br J Plast Surg. 1962;15:242–54.
74. Cox AT. The cleavage lines of the skin. Br J Surg. 1941;29:234.
75. Rubin LR. Langer's lines and facial scars. Plast Reconstr Surg. 1948;3:147–55.
76. Borges AF. Elective incisions and scar revision. Boston: Little, Brown and Company; 1973.
77. Sarifakioglu N, Terzioglu A, Ates L, et al. A new phenomenon: "sleep lines" on the face. Scand J Plast Reconstr Surg Hand Surg. 2004;38:244–7.
78. Kraissl CJ. The selection of appropriate lines for elective surgical incisions. Plast Reconstr Surg (1946). 1951;8(1):1–28.
79. Pierard GE, Lapiere CM. Microanatomy of the dermis in relation to relaxed skin tension lines and Langer's lines. Am J Dermatopathol. 1987;9:219–24.
80. Langer K. Zur Anatomie und Physiologie der Haul.III. Uber die Elasticitiit der Cutis. Sitzungsber Math Cl Kaiserlich Acad Wiss. 1862;45:156.
81. Gillespie PH, Banwell PE, Hormbrey EL, et al. A new model for assessment in plastic surgery: knowledge of relaxed skin tension lines. Br J Plast Surg. 2000;53:243–4.
82. Su CW, Alizadeh K, Lee RC. The scar problem. Clin Plast Surg. 1998;25:451.
83. Scott P, Gahary A, Chambers M, et al. Biological basis of hypertrophic scarring. Adv Struct Biol. 1994;3:157.

84. Grinell F, Zhu M, Carlson MA, Abrams JM. Release of mechanical tension triggers apoptosis of human fibroblasts in a model of regressing granulation tissue. Exp Cell Res. 1999;248:608.

85. Mustoe TA. Prevention of excessive scar formation: a surgical perspective. In: Teot L, Ziegler UE, Banwell PE, editors. Surgery in wounds. Berlin: Springer; 2004. p. 489.

86. Pierard GE, Pierard-Franchimont C, Lapiere CM. Histopathology aid at the diagnosis of the Ehlers-Danlos syndrome gravis and mitis types. Int J Dermatol. 1983;22:300–4.

87. Pierard GE. Syndrome d'Ascher et Cutis Laxa. Ann Dermatol Venereol. 1983;110:237–40.

88. Kenedi RM, Gibson T. Etude Experimentale des Tensions de la Peau dans le Corps I-fumain-Systeme de Mesure des Forces et Resultats. Rev Franc Mecan. 1962;4:121.

89. Zahouani H, Djaghloul M, Vargiolu R, Mezghani S, Mansori MEL. Contribution of human skin topography to the characterization of dynamic skin tension during senescence: morpho-mechanical approach. J Phys Conf Ser. 2014;483:1. https://doi.org/10.1088/1742-6596/483/1/012012.

90. Lawrence-Katz J. Anisotropy of Young's modulus of bone. Nature. 1980;283(5742):106.

91. Stark HL. Directional variations in the extensibility of human skin. Br J Plast Surg. 1977;30:105–14.

92. Barbenel JC. Identification of Langer's lines. In: Serup J, Jemec GBE, editors. Handbook of non-invasive methods and the skin. Boca Raton: CRC Press; 1995. p. 341–4.

93. Zahouani H. Méthodes de caractérisation de la surface cutanée. Encyclopédie Médico-Chirurgicale. Editions Scientifiques et Médicales. Paris: Elsevier SAS; 2012. p. 50–140, H-10.

94. Zahouani H, Vargiolu R. Skin line morphology: tree and branches. Editions Springer measuring the skin. sous la direction du Professeur P. AGACHE; 2005. p. 40–59.

95. Hashimoto L. New methods for surface ultrastructure. Int J Dermatol. 1974;13:357–81.

96. Gibson T, Kenedi RM, Craik JE. The mobile micro-architecture of dermal collagen: a bioengineering study. Br J Surg. 1965;52(10):764–70.

97. Morgan FR. The mechanical properties of collagen fibres-stress/strain curves. Soc Leather Tr Chem. 1960;44:170.

98. Kenedi RM, Gibson T, Daly CH. Bioengineering studies of the human skin, the effect of unidirectional tension. London: Butterworth; 1965.

99. Vogel HG. Effects of age on the biomechanical and biochemical properties of rat and human skin. J Soc Cosmet Chem. 1983;34:453–63.

100. Brown RE, Butler JP, Rogers RA, Leith DE. Mechanical connections between elastin and collagen. Connect Tissue Res. 1994;30:295.

101. Staloff IA, Guan E, Katz S, Rafailovitch M, Sokolov A, Sokolov S. An in vivo study of the mechanical properties of facial skin and influence of aging using digital image speckle correlation. Skin Res Technol. 2008;14(2):127–34.

102. Agache PG, Monneur C, Leveque JL, et al. Mechanical properties and Young's modulus of human skin in vivo. Arch Dermatol Res. 1980;269:221–32.

103. Silver F, Siperko L, Seehra G. Mechanobiology of force transduction in dermal tissue. Skin Res Technol. 2003;9:3–23.

104. Balin A, Kligman A. Aging and the skin. New York: Raven Press; 1989.

105. Wilkes G, Brown I, Wildnauer R. The biomechanical properties of skin. CRC Crit Rev Biomed. 1973;1(4):453–95.

106. Carmichael SW. The tangled web of Langer's lines. Clin Anat. 2014;27:162–8.

107. Howes EL, Harvey SC. Clinical significance of experimental studies in wound healing. Ann Surg. 1935;102:94.

108. Howes EL, Sooy J, Harvey SC. Healing of wounds as determined by their tensile strength. JAMA. 1929;92:42.

109. Capek L, Jacquet E, Dzan L, Simunek A. The analysis of forces needed for the suturing of elliptical skin wounds. Med Biol Eng Comput. 2012;50:193–8.

110. Wunderlich RC, Heerema NA. Hair crown patterns of human newborns. Studies on parietal hair whorl locations and their directions. Clin Pediatr. 1975;14(11):1045–9.
111. Tolhurst MD, Carstens MH, Greco RJ, Hurwitz DJ. The surgical anatomy of the scalp. Plast Reconstr Surg. 1991;87:603.
112. Jackson IT. General considerations. In: Jackson IT, editor. Local flaps in head and neck reconstruction. St. Louis: Mosby; 1985. p. 4–5.
113. Azzoloni A, Riberti C, Caalca D. Skin expansion in head and neck reconstructive surgery. Plast Reconstr Surg. 1992;90:799.
114. Sasaki GH. Intraoperative sustained limited expansion (ISLE) as an immediate reconstructive technique. Clin Plast Surg. 1987;14:563.
115. Camirand A, Doucet JA. Comparison between parallel hairline incisions and perpendicular incisions when performing a facelift. Plast Reconstr Surg. 1995;99:10.
116. Paul SP. Rotation flaps of the scalp: study of the design, planning and biomechanics of single, double and triple pedicle flaps. In: Paul SP, Norman RA, editors. Clinical cases in skin cancer surgery and treatment, clinical cases in dermatology. Basel: Springer; 2016. p. 31–44.
117. Cutting C. Critical closing and perfusion pressures in flap survival. Ann Plast Surg. 1982;9:524.
118. Topaz M, Carmel NN, Topaz G, Li M, Li YZ. Stress–relaxation and tension relief system for immediate primary closure of large and huge soft tissue defects: an old–new concept: new concept for direct closure of large defects. Medicine. 2014;93(28):e234.
119. Raposio E, Nordström RE. Biomechanical properties of scalp flaps and their correlations to reconstructive and aesthetic surgery procedures. Skin Res Technol. 1998;4:94–8.
120. Paul SP, Matulich J, Charlton NA. New skin tensiometer device: computational analyses to understand biodynamic excisional skin tension lines. Sci Rep. 2016;6:30117. https://doi.org/10.1038/srep30117.
121. Paul SP. The keystone design perforator island flap: an easy option for the lower limb, but how does it actually work? In: Paul SP, Norman RA, editors. Clinical cases in skin cancer surgery and treatment, clinical cases in dermatology. Basel: Springer; 2016. p. 65–79.
122. Behan FC, Terrill PJ, Breidahl A, Cavallo A, Ashton M. Island flaps including the Bezier type in the treatment of malignant melanoma. Aust N Z J Surg. 1995;65:870–80.
123. Taylor GI, Doyle M, McCarten G. The Doppler probe for planning flaps: anatomical study and clinical applications. Br J Plast Surg. 1990;43:1–16.
124. Behan FC. The keystone design perforator island flap in reconstructive surgery. ANZ J Surg. 2003;73:112–20.
125. Behan FC, Lo C. Principles and misconceptions regarding the keystone island flap. Ann Surg Oncol. 2009;16:1722–3.
126. Milton SH. Experimental studies on island flaps. Plast Reconstr Surg. 1972;48(6):574–8.
127. Jordan DJ, Malahias M, Hindocha S, Juma A. Flap decisions and options in soft tissue coverage of the lower limb. Open Orthop J. 2014;8:423–32.
128. Haertsch PA. The surgical plane in the leg. Br J Plast Surg. 1981;34:464–9.
129. Douglas CD, Low NC, Seitz MJ. The 'keystone concept': time for some science. Perspectives ANZ J Surg. 2013;83:498–504.
130. Douglas CD, Low NC, Seitz MJ. The keystone flap: not an advance, just a stretch. Ann Surg Oncol. 2013;20:973–80.
131. Leshin B, Whitaker DC, Swanson NA. An approach to patient assessment and preparation in cutaneous oncology. J Am Acad Dermatol. 1988;19:1081–8.
132. Balch CM, Milton GW, Shaw HM, Seng-Jaw S. Cutaneous melanoma. Philadelphia: JB Lippincott; 1985. p. 71–90.
133. Bennett RG. Fundamentals of cutaneous surgery. St. Louis: CV Mosby; 1988. p. 353–44.
134. Leshin B. Proper planning and execution of surgical excisions. Chapter 15: Basic surgical concepts and procedures. In: Wheeland RG, editor. Cutaneous surgery. Philadelphia: WB Saunders; 1994. p. 171–7.

135. Bernstein L. Incisions and excisions in elective facial surgery. Arch Otolaryngol. 1973;97:238–43.
136. Pinkus F. Die Faltung der Haut. In: Pinkus F, editor. Die normale Anatomie der Haut. Jadassohn's Handbuch der Haut und Geschlechtskrankheiten, vol. 1. Berlin: Springer; 1927. p. 4–76.
137. Pinkus F. Die Faltung der Haut. In: Pinkus F, editor. Die normale Anatomie der Haut. Jadassohn's Handbuch der Haut und Geschlechtskrankheiten, vol. 1. Berlin: Springer; 1927. p. 4–76.
138. Paul SP. Biodynamic excisional skin tension (BEST) lines: revisiting Langer's lines, skin biomechanics, current concepts in cutaneous surgery, and the (lack of) science behind skin lines used for surgical excisions. J Dermatol Res. 2017;2(1):77–87.

Chapter 2
Why the Geological Approach Doesn't Work for Wrinkles: The Need to Move from Anatomy to Physiology

During 2010–2011 in New Zealand, where this author is based, the Canterbury region suffered a major earthquake, and many faults were identified in the landscape [1]. All these newly discovered faults raised questions as to how many of these had been missed previously. Walls of active normal faults typically form a series of sub-basins separated by intra-basin highs. These intra-basin highs commonly expose hanging wall basements in direct contact with the footwall, whereas hanging wall basements on either side of intra-basin highs are buried by basin landfills [2]. It is generally accepted that intra-basin highs mark locations where two originally isolated fault segments linked together [2].

Geological folds or anticlines were first identified in the 1860s, during the same period when Karl Langer published his treatise on skin tension lines [3]. The prevailing theory was that these faults were sine-wave-like folds resulting from compression of the sedimentary section over a yielding substrate with no involvement of basement or underlying rocks and no underlying faults [4]. Dahlstrom developed the theory of "balanced cross-sections", where in a geological cross-section, one flattens out the deformed beds and returns them to their original horizontal position [5]. Others have commented that it is the resistance to forward movement of the layers in front that causes rocks to bend upward in an asymmetric fashion. This movement gives rise to shortening of the beds across the structure as the area becomes horizontally compressed [4].

Folds have long been recognized as important structural traps from a geological point of view. Fault-parallel folds, such as drag-folds and rollover-folds form because of movement on the associated normal fault systems [6] and these are like what we observe during skin wrinkling. In addition to variations in fault displacements, displacement also decreases with distance normal to the fault surface, resulting in a reverse-drag geometry in both the hanging wall and footwall [7]. Ultimately, as Schlische notes, maximum displacement occurs at the center of the fault and decreases toward the fault tips; displacement decreases with distance from the fault surface; faults increase in length as displacement increases; and fault systems are commonly segmented [8]—not unlike what we observe in what happens to wrinkle

© Springer International Publishing AG, part of Springer Nature 2018
S. P. Paul, *Biodynamic Excisional Skin Tension Lines for Cutaneous Surgery*,
https://doi.org/10.1007/978-3-319-71495-0_2

lines of skin during an elliptical excision where maximum tension and displacement occurs in the middle and decreases towards the tips.

According to Van Elst [9], there are three types of faults that result in earthquakes: strike-slip, normal and thrust (reverse) faults, and each type is the outcome of different forces pushing or pulling on the crust, causing rocks to slide up, down or past each other.

When studies were done on mice, exposing them to UV-B radiation for 10 weeks, their skin showed spontaneous contraction in response to UV irradiation. Wrinkled skin showed a marked decrease in the wrinkle depth and a slight increase in wrinkle interval following muscle layer removal, a unique deformation that cannot be explained if homogeneity is applied to skin deformation [9]. Matsumoto developed a model for what occurs during UV-induced damage on skin: spontaneous contraction of the dermis while maintaining or increasing the epidermal area induces buckling of the epidermis into the dermis at mechanically weak lines. Where rows of pores and sulci exist, buckling becomes amplified by the axial compression of the dermis by the muscle layer [10]. We can also predict biomechanical wrinkling based on morphology i.e. observations show that wrinkles coincide with rows of pores and sulci cutis, i.e. the areas where the structural stiffness of the horny layer is relatively low [10].

While we can note similarities when we apply geological principles to wrinkle lines, we must note that not all wrinkles are created equal. Bosset and others studied the clinical and histopathological features of permanent and reducible wrinkles [11]. Noting that not enough research had been done into wrinkling and skin folds, this team analyzed the histological features of the pre-auricular wrinkles and compared this to retro-auricular skin from patients undergoing cutaneous surgery to the face. The skin samples were immediately processed for routine histology and histochemical staining. Based on these observations, skin depressions were classified into four types according to their depth: folds, permanent wrinkles, reducible wrinkles and skin micro-relief [11].

Bosset et al. [11] further divided wrinkles as follows: (1) permanent wrinkles which were conserved after sampling and (2) reducible wrinkles which required *in vivo* staining to be visible at histology. We now begin to appreciate that treating all wrinkles similarly is unscientific, especially their use as excisional lines (as opposed to using them for surgical egress). Bosset and team concluded that both types of wrinkles were made up of skin modifications—in the upper dermis, permanent wrinkles had a more pronounced accumulation of basophilic fibres, i.e. actinic elastosis, than reducible wrinkles did. They felt that the development of wrinkles could be secondary to actinic elastosis—due to the disappearance of microfibrils and collagen fibres at the dermal-epidermal junction [11].

In 2003, Cerda and Mahadevan [12] studied the physics and geometry of membrane wrinkling—they took a food-grade plastic sheet, cut ribbons from the middle and stretched the sheet. They noted that wrinkles appeared parallel to the ribbon, and the wavelength (λ) was proportional to the square root of the sample size. They then extrapolated their research to human skin. They noted that human wrinkling is generally more notable where there is excess skin (such as the backs of hands) or where skin is close to bone (such as the forehead or crow's feet).

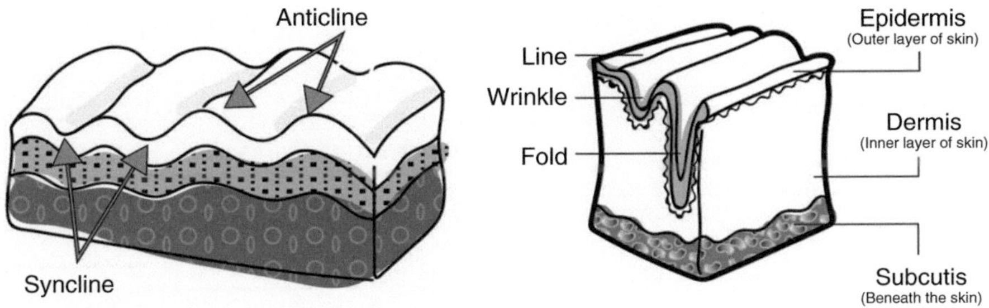

Fig. 2.1 Comparing the folds on the Earth's crust and the human cutis

If human skin is viewed as a mere physical membrane, wrinkles fundamentally occur because a keratinocyte-stiffened epidermis drapes a softer and thicker dermis. Of course anatomical sites like knees and elbows have wrinkles that can be considered 'tension' wrinkles (two-dimensional, due to geometry, pre-tension and joint action) and in other areas like the forehead, muscle action causes 'compression' wrinkles (one-dimensional due to muscle action only).

The author has been fascinated by the concept of wrinkles and relaxed skin tension lines being used as surgical guidelines, given these have become widely adopted with no conclusive scientific basis—and both types of lines differ in direction, yet are considered acceptable for surgical incisions. In animals such as pigs, for example, with age and fat deposition skin tension lines begin to run transversely, whereas in thinner animals, skin tension lines run more obliquely [13]. To get a better understanding of any condition, it is better to study its loss or excess. In 2010 [14], there was a report of a Japanese baby with Michelin Tyre Baby Syndrome, a condition that causes folding of excess skin. However, as was noted in this case report, in some babies with this syndrome spontaneous recovery occurs i.e. wrinkles simply disappear. Most notably, skin fold biopsies from these babies showed no epidermal, dermal or subcutaneous tissue abnormalities. Surely there must be an underlying anatomical reason why wrinkles occur?

Geologically speaking, folds occurring in the Earth's 'skin' are conceptually no different to wrinkles on any multi-layered surface. These geological folds occur when flat and stacked planar surfaces, such as sedimentary strata, are bent or curved as a result of permanent deformations. To the author, geological folds seem epistemologically related to cutaneous folds, as illustrated in the figure (Fig. 2.1). Berg [15] proposed a model for anticline formation—showing that ranges became raised along a partially listric, sub-horizontal thrust fault. However, this model showed the down-dip portion of the fault plunging at depth, which was only possible if basement rocks were plastic and therefore later discredited [4]. Later, geologists adopted the model of 'balanceable cross sections' [4]. On observing the anticline formations in old rocks, it appears that it is the resistance to forward movement of the layers in front which causes the rocks to bend upward in an asymmetric fashion, causing wrinkling. Anticlines occur in old rocks just as wrinkling occurs in aging skin. These geological 'compression' wrinkles gives rise to shortening of the beds across

Fig. 2.2 From: The
Anatomical Basis for
wrinkles showing a
lymphatic vessel under
each wrinkle (From Pessa
et al. Aesthet Surg J. 2014;
34: 2, 227–234 with
permission)

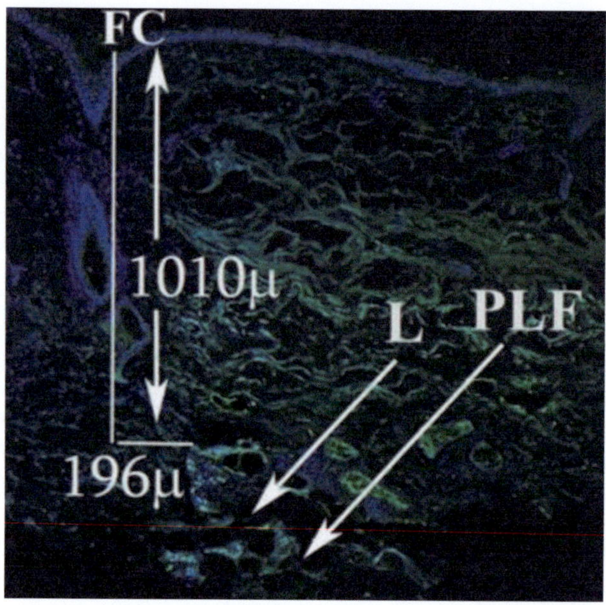

the structure as the area becomes horizontally compressed, not dissimilar conceptually to the formation of cutaneous wrinkles with age. However, there was one matter unresolved—geologically there are differences notable in the underlying strata,—but histologically, as we discussed in the "Michelin Tyre Baby" case above, there was no underlying differences noted on anatomic pathology examination.

Pessa and others set out to answer this question—is there an underlying anatomical basis for wrinkles—can biology follow geology? Pessa studied creases such as crow's feet, and forehead wrinkles [16]. They found that each and every wrinkle they studied occurred within ±1 mm of a major lymphatic vessel and its surrounding tube of adipose tissue. They concluded that an anatomical basis for wrinkles does exist and these are lymphatic vessels, along with the surrounding distinct perilymphatic fat, present directly beneath wrinkles and creases [16]. The forehead crease in the image (Fig. 2.2) lies 196 μm lateral to a main lymphatic vessel (L) and its perilymphatic fat (PLF). The speckling indicates the presence of antigens associated with lymphatic vessels, in this case podoplanin and PROX1.

This may have implications for surgery. Until recently, incisions were planned in wrinkle or crease lines with the theory being as collagen runs parallel to wrinkle lines, collagen will be laid down in the same direction as is normal within wrinkle lines and the septa between skin and muscle—leaving to the best possible scars. However, the author's group recently noted that incisional and excisional lines are different i.e. when skin is excised and tension created, as is done after skin cancer surgery, different dynamics apply and wrinkle lines no longer have the least wound tension [17].

More recently, it has come to light that wrinkles can be caused due to aging and oxidative stress—and indeed increased wrinkling may be a sign of impending heart disease, metabolic disorders, osteoporosis or degenerative disorders [18]. And, while photo-damage from sunlight is one of the most common causes in Caucasian skin, recent studies have shown that UV light also damages lymphatic channels [19]. Some of the genetic mechanisms behind wrinkling are disturbed lipid metabolism, altered insulin and STAT3 signaling, upregulation of apoptotic genes partly due to the deregulation of FOXO1, downregulation of members of the jun and fos family, differential expression of cytoskeletal proteins (e.g., keratin 2A, 6A, and 16A), extracellular matrix components (e.g., PI3, S100A2, A7, A9, SPRR2B), and proteins involved in cell-cycle control (e.g., CDKs, GOS2) [20].

The direct finding of an anatomical relationship between lymphatic channels and wrinkles is a good direction for new research. This has implications for not only surgical lines, but also in understanding why chronic illness or cancer often accelerates the aging process. Tybjærg-Hansen and others studied over 10,000 Danes and found that ear lobe creases indicated the body's biological age, and was an indicator for heart disease [21]. Studies on Shar Pei dogs suggest these animals have mucinosis—high hyaluronic acid levels are found in both cutaneous tissues and the blood stream—and these high amounts are due to an excess in the activity (overexpression) of the HAS2 enzyme [22]. Such research avenues are promising as they can shed more light on processes such as cell recognition and ageing.

Therefore, when it comes to wrinkles, beauty may indeed be more than skin-deep. Kraissl favoured wrinkle lines for surgical excisions [23]. Kraissl himself noted these were for "small" surgical incisions. Further, Kraissl only suggested them for the facial region, where the prominent SMAS (superficial musculo-aponeurotic system) layer gives the facial skin different properties from truncal skin.

We now know that there are many different types of wrinkles, and that under each permanent wrinkle lies a lymphatic vessel. Pre-mature aging of skin and earlobe creases have been considered markers of systemic disease and therefore we do not yet know if using wrinkle lines for excision of large tumours, especially those prone to lymphatic spread, can make things worse due to the increased tension an excision creates [24]. As the author has noted in other articles, surgical practice when it comes to wrinkle lines seems to adopt a geological or topographical approach, ignoring the underlying physiology [24]. Fundamentally, wrinkle lines are folds not designed to be excisional lines except possibly for very small skin lesions and in the following chapters we will discuss biodynamic excisional skin tension (BEST) lines and why closing the wound under least tension (along BEST lines) allows for the best outcomes.

References

1. Jongens R, Barrell DJA, Campbell JK, Pettinga JR. Faulting and folding beneath the Canterbury Plains identified prior to the 2010 emergence of the Greendale Fault. N Z J Geol Geophys. 2012;55(3):169–76.
2. Anders M, Schlische R. Overlapping faults, intrabasin highs, and the growth of normal faults. J Geol. 1994;102(2):165–79.

3. Langer K. Zur Anatomie und Physiologie der Haut. Über die Spaltbarkeit der Cutis. Sitzungsbericht der Mathematisch-naturwissenschaftlichen Classe der Wiener Kaiserlichen Academie der Wissenschaften 1861, Abt 44.
4. Parkar Gay S Jr. New advancements in understanding the formation of anticlines. 2012. http://www.appliedgeophysics.com/images/understanding-anticlines.pdf. Accessed 1 Aug 2016.
5. Dahlstrom CDA. Balanced cross sections. Can J Earth Sci. 1969;6:743–57.
6. Hamblin WK. Origin of "reverse drag" on the down-thrown sides of normal faults. Bull Geol Soc Am. 1965;76:1145–64.
7. Barnett JAM, Mortimer J, Rippon JH, Walsh JJ, Watterson J. Displacement geometry in the volume containing a single normal fault. AAPG Bull. 1987;71:925–37.
8. Schlische RW. Geometry and origin of fault-related folds in extensional settings. AAPG Bull. 1995;79(11):1661–78.
9. Van Elst N quoted by Oskin B in "Fault lines: facts about cracks in the earth." Live Sci. 25 Sept 2014. https://www.livescience.com/37052-types-of-faults.html. Accessed 15 Aug 2017.
10. Matsumoto T. Biomechanics of wrinkle formation. J Jpn Cosmet Sci Soc. 2013;37(2):101–6.
11. Bosset S, Barre P, Chalon A, et al. Skin ageing: clinical and histopathologic study of permanent and reducible wrinkles. Eur J Dermatol. 2002;12(3):247–52.
12. Cerda E, Mahadevan L. Geometry and physics of wrinkling. Phys Rev Lett. 2003;90(7):0743021–3.
13. Rose EH, Vistnes LM, Ksander VA. Skin tension lines in the domestic pig. Plast Reconstr Surg. 1977;59(2):269–71.
14. Nomura Y, Ota M, Tochimaru H. Self-healing congenital generalized skin creases: Michelin tire baby syndrome. J Am Acad Dermatol. 2010;63(6):1110–1.
15. Berg RR. Mountain flank thrusting in Rocky Mountain foreland, Wyoming and Colorado. AAPG Bull. 1962;46:2019–32.
16. Pessa JE, Nguyen H, John GB, Scherer PE. The anatomical basis for wrinkles. Aesthet Surg J. 2014;34(2):227–34.
17. Paul SP, Matulich J, Charlton N. A new skin tensiometer device: computational analyses to understand biodynamic excisional skin tension lines. Sci Rep. 2016;6:30117.
18. Makrantonaki E, Bekou V, Zouboulis CC. Genetics and skin aging. Dermato-Endocrinology. 2012;4(3):280–4.
19. Kajiya K, Kunstfeld R, Chung JH, Detmar M. Reduction of lymphatic vessels in photodamaged skin. J Dermatol Sci. 2007;47:241–3.
20. Lener T, Moll PR, Rinnerthaler M, Bauer J, Aberger F, Richter K. Expression profiling of aging in the human skin. Exp Gerontol. 2006;41(4):387–97.
21. Christoffersen M, Frikke-Schmidt R, Schnohr P, Jensen GB, Nordestgaard BG, Tybjærg-Hansen A. Visible age-related signs and risk of ischemic heart disease in the general population: a prospective cohort study. Circulation. 2014;129(9):990–8.
22. Universitat Autònoma de Barcelona. Why Shar Pei dogs have so many wrinkles. ScienceDaily. 16 Nov 2008. https://www.sciencedaily.com/releases/2008/11/081111163123.htm. Accessed 15 Aug 2017.
23. Kraissl CJ, Conway H. Excision of small tumors of the skin of the face with special reference to the wrinkle lines. Surgery. 1949;25:592.
24. Paul SP. The epistemology of wrinkles: from geology and anatomy to physiology. Int J Biomed. 2016;6(3):237–9.

Chapter 3
Understanding the Interplay Between Elastin and Collagen During Surgical Procedures and Their Relationship to BEST Lines

Previously, surgeons have not differentiated between incisional and excisional skin tension—or considered the notion that planning of incisions during excisional surgery may be different from surgery for egress. Skin is after all a composite material that comprises a fibrous network within a ground substance [1]. It has been well known among students of biomechanics that at low loads, skin is more compliant in the axial direction than in the transverse, and skin relaxes much faster in the axial direction than in the transverse direction [2]. In contrast to healthy skin, scars relax faster because of their higher viscous content and therefore scars have reduced ability to handle load, displacement and energy—indicating they do not have the burst strength, extensibility, and toughness of uninjured skin [3]. Prior research into hypertrophic scars has shown that in these scars, high-load linear stiffness is relatively unaffected, whereas low-loads exhibit a more dramatic response—indicating that the interplay between elastin and collagen is different between low-loads and high-loads of skin tension [4].

Pigs have been a good clinical model for the study of wounds and scars because they are structurally and functionally like human skin [5]. Others have even suggested that different breeds of pig exhibit responses to wounding that parallel those observed among humans of different ethnicities [3]! However, biomechanical studies generally give us insight only into the viscoelastic properties relevant to physiologic use and tissue failure properties, but do not give us good insight into the interplay between collagen and elastin and hence this investigation was designed to see what happened to collagen and elastin during skin incisions and excisions.

3.1 Anatomical Structure of Elastin and Collagen

It has been known that orienting scars differently can have different outcomes. A cadaver study noted the unequal distributions of dermal collagen and elastin in skin sections perpendicular to each other from different regions of the body [6].

© Springer International Publishing AG, part of Springer Nature 2018
S. P. Paul, *Biodynamic Excisional Skin Tension Lines for Cutaneous Surgery*,
https://doi.org/10.1007/978-3-319-71495-0_3

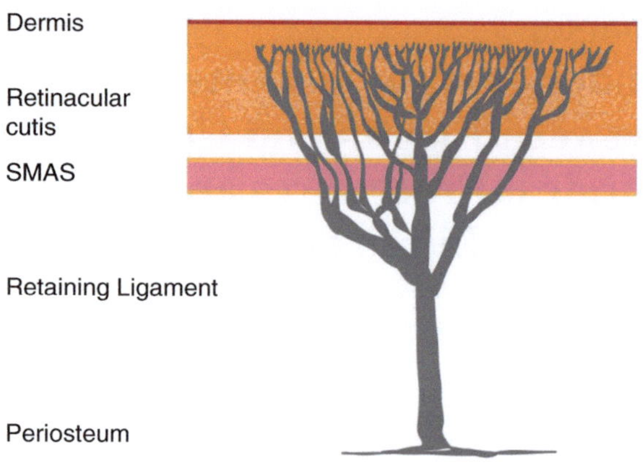

Fig. 3.1 The structure of the skin and ligamentous attachments can be likened to a tree

The authors noted that this unequal distribution would affect the wound healing process that in turn could cause varied scar appearance and behaviour depending on the region and direction of wound [6].

The term "Apophänie" was coined by Klaus Conrad to describe early stages of schizophrenia—the unmotivated seeing of connections and attributing abnormal meaningfulness [7, 8]. In medicine we often exhibit apophenic tendencies, making connections between unrelated things—"anchovy sauce" pus of an amoebic liver abscess, "arborizing" or tree-like vessels that are noted in the dermoscopy of a basal cell cancer and "strawberry" angiomas. Pareidolia is a type of apophenia involving the perception of images in random places and in this context, skin and connective tissue structure of the face can be likened to a tree (Fig. 3.1). Because of the presence of the SMAS (superficial musculo-aponeurotic layer) the face needs unique considerations. Other authors have also suggested that the ligaments of the fibrous support system of the face can be likened to a tree. The retaining ligaments are attached to the periosteum and deep muscle fascia and fan out via a series of branches into and through the SMAS. In the outer part of the subcutaneous layer, the increased number of progressively finer retinacular cutis fibres securely attach themselves to the dermis [9].

Elastin is a protein and a major part of the extracellular matrix of connective tissue. Elastin molecules are configured in a three-dimensional network, rather like rubber—and similarly elastin can be stretched to 2.5 times the length of the unloaded configuration [10]. Collagen is also a protein and can be considered the main load bearing element in a wide variety of tissues. In tissues like the Achilles Tendon that are high load-bearing, it must be noted that collagen is 20 times as prevalent as elastin. In contrast, the ligamentum nuchae contains five times as much elastin as collagen. A third of amino acids in both collagen and elastin consist of glycine. However, the proline and hydroxyproline contents are much lower in elastin than in collagen molecules [10]. In contrast to hard tissues, soft tissues like skin and connective tissue exhibit viscoelastic behavior such as relaxation and creep, which have been associated with the interaction of collagen with the matrix of proteoglycans [11]. The concept of tissue expansion is an important method of wound closure in plastic surgery and is essentially based on understanding the skin's ability to "creep". During tissue expansion, acute tension is applied to the skin leading to elongation followed by relaxation and retraction to exceed its initial length. Following repeated stress-relaxation, the skin may elongate permanently to a limited extent [12].

When considering creep, it must be noted that beyond skin creep and surgical technique, suture materials also demonstrate a degree of suture creep and this ends up a third confounding variable in cutaneous surgery. A study was conducted comparing creep measurements of 0 and 2-0 Prolene (Ethicon, Johnson & Johnson Intl., Somerville, NJ) and 1 and 2-0 PDSII (Ethicon, Johnson & Johnson Intl.) sutures. Two different loads were used representing normal intra-abdominal pressure (IAP). This study showed that different suture materials exhibited different degrees of creep. All suture materials showed significant (3–51%) creep behaviour. Prolene sutures showed more creep than PDSII sutures in both loading conditions [13]. Further discussion regarding the creep of suture materials is beyond the scope of this article which will concentrate on elastin, collagen and skin creep.

Elastin, as the name indicates, makes skin elastic—providing the organ with the ability to stretch and recoil [14]. Collagen in skin responds to mechanical forces by altering its molecular structure and generates biochemical signals to influence wound healing and tissue remodelling [15]. Levels of collagen and elastin change with the depth of the dermis and age—and in the lower dermis a significant difference between young and old has been noted for elastin with varying collagen/elastin ratios [16]. Since Langer's seminal work in 1861, his 'cleavage lines of skin' ended up de facto surgical lines, even for most surgical excisions of skin lesions [17, 18]. It has already been suggested by others that in the trunk and limbs, Langer's lines predominantly align with elastin fibres [19].

After Langer marked out cleavage lines by using a round-tipped cutting instrument and noting the direction the clefts elongated, Kocher, in 1892, suggested that these lines be used for surgical procedures [20]. It has been noted in recent times that incisions placed at right angles to the direction of skin cleavage lines had a higher risk of haematoma and tension, and thereby a higher risk of hypertrophic scarring [21]. But the mechanisms of wound tension, especially when defects are created due to the removal of skin lesions have been poorly understood. Biomechanical studies have shown that skin behaves elastically only at low-load levels. For example, on the feet, due to weight-bearing tissues where the load increases, skin reveals increased viscoelastic behavior, i.e. strain becomes a function of load and time [22]. While it is well known that skin is anisotropic, it also exhibits orthotropy i.e. a degree of symmetry with regard to two normal planes, especially in regions of the body close to bone [23]. One of the theories has been that this is due to a preferential orientation of collagen fibres [24].

Incisions made along the long-axis of skin cleavage lines are essentially lines in the direction of minimum skin extensibility, and in areas like the calf, 76% of elastin fibres aligned themselves along Langer's lines [25]. Yet, we know from other studies

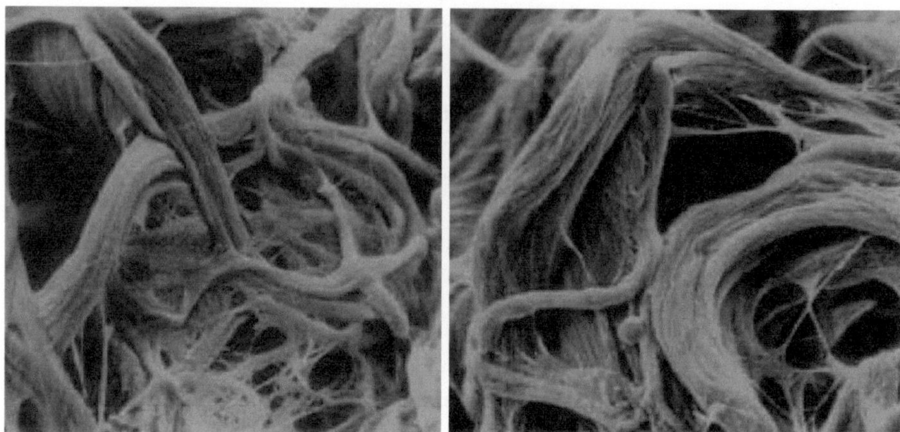

Fig. 3.2 Normal skin: collagen and elastin. Reprinted with permission from "Microanatomy of the Dermis in Relation to Relaxed Skin Tension Lines and Langer's Lines." Piérard, GE; Lapière. American Journal of Dermatopathology: June 1987 (SEM. (a) ×230; (b) ×460; (c) ×930; (d) ×1100)

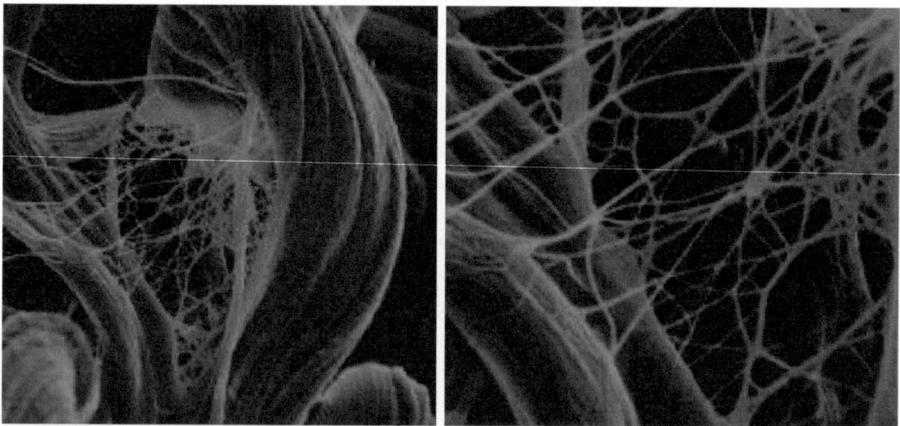

Fig. 3.3 Interplay between collagen and elastin during surgery. Adapted and reprinted with permission from "Microanatomy of the Dermis in Relation to Relaxed Skin Tension Lines and Langer's Lines." Piérard, GE; Lapière. American Journal of Dermatopathology: June 1987

that in the superficial dermis, collagen fibres are not oriented along cleavage lines and it is the reticular dermis that determines skin anisotropy [26]. It is clear that the interplay between elastin and collagen (Figs. 3.2 and 3.3) is a major influence on scarring and wound behaviour.

However, the precise roles of elastin and collagen during skin stretch or load for excisional surgery have been unknown until now. In this chapter, the author investigates incisional and excisional skin wounds to try and understand if the roles of elastin and collagen under low- and high-tension loads differ.

3.2   Materials and Methods

For this study, the author used a two-photon microscopic camera using optimal wavelengths to detect collagen and elastin. Previous studies have detected collagen and elastin in skin using fluorescence imaging using specific emission wavelengths: lambda c for collagen at 380 nm, and for elastin 450 nm, using excitation wavelengths (lambda e) of 340 and 380 nm, respectively [27]. These parameters were used as a guide in planning this study. A study was undertaken in five patients (n = 5; age range 25–74) who were undergoing cutaneous surgery for skin cancer. Measurements were taken at the center of the "excisional" wound (high-load) and at the ends of the wound (tapered end of the ellipse) where effectively the wound is an "incisional" wound.

Using a two-photon microscopic camera (developed in house in conjunction with Shenzhen Do3think Technology Co., Ltd) measurements were taken of incisional and excisional sites in each case (Fig. 3.4).

Under a spectroscope, elastin is similar to collagen with an absorption peak around 320 nm and an emission peak near 400 nm. Collagen can similarly be viewed using a SHG microscopic camera where two photons combine from the

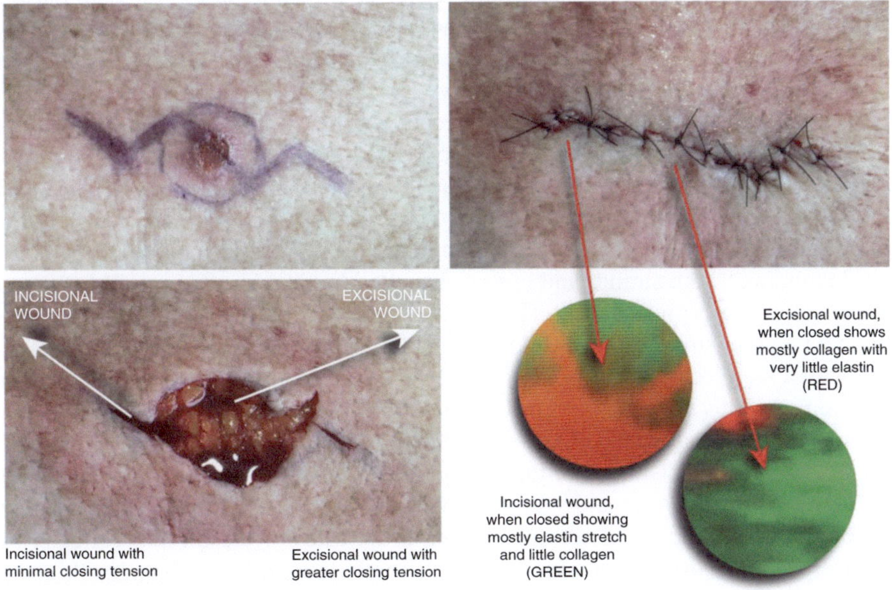

Fig. 3.4 Interplay between collagen and elastin when viewed under two-photon microscopy

laser field to produce a scattered photon of exactly half the wavelength [28]. The study showed second-harmonic generation signals derived from collagen can be spectrally isolated from elastin two-photon fluorescence. Two-photon fluorescence signals can be further characterized by emission maxima at 495 and 520 nm, corresponding to elastin and cellular contributions. This method may not be strictly fluorescence, but is very useful to visualize collagen and elastin separately. Others have also noted second-harmonic generation microscopy has emerged as a powerful modality for imaging fibrillar collagen in a diverse range of tissues, including skin [29]. Alongside confocal microscopy, two-photon microscopy is now also being used to detect skin cancer and some authors have successfully used this method to monitor collagen remodelling *in vivo* after micro-ablative fractional laser resurfacing [30].

3.3 Results

Wounds were observed *after* they were surgically closed as shown in the image. When incisional wounds were observed, where there was minimal tension (<1.5 N force) we found that in each case elastin stretched and collagen buckled, revealing mostly elastin. Where larger defects were created after excisions (as in the figure where a skin cancer had been removed, where forces to close wound were typically greater than 2 N), we noted the image revealed mostly collagen, suggesting the reverse occurred i.e. collagen stretched and elastin buckled.

Multi-photon microscopy has found favour as a technique to elucidate elastin and collagen in tissues [31]. The main advantage of multi-photon microscopy is based on two-photon excited fluorescence (TPEF) and second harmonic generation (SHG) imaging—allowing us to observe non-fixed, unstained tissue samples. Because collagen in the skin dermis can easily produce a SHG signal and elastin is more effective in generating TPEF, -photon microscopy has found widespread applications in dermatology for studying and differentiating cutaneous collagen and elastin—in general using this technique the collagen images are colour-coded in green and elastin images are colour-coded in red to increase the contrast [31, 32].

The findings were similar and in fact virtually identical in *all cases*. The images demonstrating a typical finding (Fig. 3.3) show for incisional lines (low tension wounds) elastin stretches and collagen buckles, and for excisional wounds (after removal of skin lesions) it is predominantly collagen at play with very little elastin involvement. This not only confirms the author's contention regarding biodynamic excisional skin tension (BEST) lines [33] that we must view skin lines differently for incisions and excisions, but the author sees this as the starting point for more research into wound, scar and skin dynamics after excisional surgery. This was the reason for the enquiry that set out to look at the roles of elastin and collagen in surgical wounds when closing incisions (inherently low-load) or excisions (higher-loads due to larger defects).

The author's finding that incisional (low-load) wound closures are primarily under the influence of elastin, and excisional wound (higher-load) closures depend on collagen has implications for research into both wound healing, suture-placement and scar formation.

3.4 Discussion

This difference between tension loads on skin and the interplay between collagen and elastin has never before been elucidated between incisional and excisional wounds, and in the author's view has great research interest for a cutaneous surgeon seeking to identify the best skin lines to utilise to minimise scarring. However, until now there has been no attempt to differentiate incisional and excisional skin lines.

The author's hypothesis that we need to view incisional and excisional wounds differently led to the mapping of best excisional skin tension (BEST) lines [20]. Human skin, when viewed as a mere physical membrane ends up with skin lines and wrinkles because a keratinocyte-stiffened epidermis drapes a softer and thicker dermis. Of course, anatomical sites like knees and elbows have wrinkles that can be considered 'tension' wrinkles (two-dimensional, due to geometry, pre-tension and joint action) and in other areas like forehead, muscle action causes 'compression' wrinkles (one-dimensional due to muscle action only), but in the author's view, BEST lines for surgical excisions may not be along these lines [34]. Add to this, others' findings that in keloid scars the increase of both elastin and collagen occurs in deep dermis, whereas a sharp decrease of elastin is found in the upper dermis of keloid [35]—and we have the beginnings of new insights and research into cutaneous surgery and wound healing.

Keloids are unique to humans with no comparable animal models [16]. Researchers have found significant differences in the morphology and content of collagen and elastin in the upper dermis and deep dermis of keloid tissue. In the upper dermis, elastin is not very visible and in the lower dermis, elastin is abundant. Given the findings in this study that incisional wounds are full of elastin and excisional wounds are filled with collagen, further avenues for research into skin lines used during surgery and the resultant scars beckon. We also know from studies into aging that changes in the functional depth of the dermis are significant only for elastin for both young and old [16]. The lower dermis is less rich in elastin and shows significant diminution between young and older age groups [16]. This also has implications for suture placement in incisional and excisional wounds. This author's studies, previously published, used multi-photon microscopy for assessing the morphology and quantity variations of collagen and elastin in incisional and excisional wounds [36], a technique used by others to study keloid scarring [31], and that is a starting point for further research to understand the basic science behind the surgical wounds we create and the resultant scar formation—as ultimately, it is the latter that patients worry about the most. This author therefore contends that incisional and excisional skin tension lines are biomechanically different and therefore understanding the interplay between elastin and collagen during surgical procedures will be of great importance for suture placement during cutaneous surgery in the future [36].

References

1. Lanir Y. Skin mechanics. In: Skalak R, Chien S, editors. Handbook of bioengineering. Dallas: McGraw-Hill; 1987. p. 11.1–11.25.
2. Corr DT, Hart DA. Biomechanics of scar tissue and uninjured skin. Adv Wound Care. 2013;2(2):37–44.
3. Corr DT, Gallant-Behm CL, Shrive NG, Hart DA. Biomechanical behavior of scar tissue and uninjured skin in a porcine model. Wound Repair Regen. 2009;17:250.
4. Dunn MG, Silver FH, Swann DA. Mechanical analysis of hypertrophic scar tissue: structural basis for apparent increased rigidity. J Invest Dermatol. 1985;8:9.
5. Gallant-Behm CL, Reno C, Tsao H, Hart DA. Genetic involvement in skin wound healing and scarring in domestic pigs: assessment of molecular expression patterns in (Yorkshire x Red Duroc) x Yorkshire backcross animals. J Invest Dermatol. 2007;127:233.
6. Kumar N, Nayak BS, Kumar P, Prasad KA. Histological study on the distribution of dermal collagen and elastic fibres in different regions of the body. Int J Med Sci. 2012;4(8):171–6.
7. Conrad K. Die beginnende Schizophrenie. Versuch einer Gestaltanalyse des Wahns [The onset of schizophrenia: an attempt to form an analysis of delusion] (in German). Stuttgart: Georg Thieme; 1958.
8. Mishara A. Klaus Conrad (1905–1961): delusional mood, psychosis and beginning schizophrenia. Schizophr Bull. 2010;36(1):9–13.
9. Mendelson B. Chapter 6: Facelift anatomy, SMAS, retaining ligaments and facial spaces. In: Aston SJ, Steinbrech DS, Walden JL, editors. Aesthetic plastic surgery. Philadelphia: Saunders, Elsevier; 2013. p. 80.
10. Holzapfel GA. Biomechanics of soft tissue. In: Lemaitre J, editor. Handbook of material behavior: nonlinear models and properties. Austria: Graz University of Technology; 2000.
11. Minns RJ, Soden PD, Jackson DS. The role of the fibrous components and ground substance in the mechanical properties of biological tissues: a preliminary investigation. J Biomech. 1973;6:153–65.
12. Topaz M. External tissue expansion and tension relief systems for improved utilisation of the viscoelastic properties of the skin in wound closure. Indian J Plast Surg. 2014;47(3):467–8.
13. Nout E, Lange JF, Salu NE, et al. Creep behavior of commonly used suture materials in abdominal wall surgery. J Surg Res. 2007;138(1):51–5.
14. Almine JF, Bax DV, Mithieux SM, Nivison-Smith L, Rnjak J, Waterhouse A, Wise SG, Weiss AS. Elastin-based materials. Chem Soc Rev. 2010;39(9):3371.
15. Chang S-W, Buehler MJ. Molecular biomechanics of collagen molecules. Mater Today. 2014;17:2.
16. Pittet J-C, Freis O, Vazquez-Duchêne M-D, Périé G, Pauly G. Evaluation of elastin/collagen content in human dermis in-vivo by multiphoton tomography—variation with depth and correlation with aging. Cosmetics. 2014;1:211–21.
17. Langer K. On the anatomy and physiology of the skin I. The cleavability of the cutis. Br J Plast Surg. 1978;31:3–8.
18. Waldorf JC, Perdikis G, Terkonda SP. Planning incisions. Oper Tech Gen Surg. 2002;4(3): 199–206.

19. Zahouani H, Djaghloul M, Vargiolu R, Mezghani S, Mansori MEL. Contribution of human skin topography to the characterization of dynamic skin tension during senescence: morpho-mechanical approach. J Phys Conf Ser. 2014;483(1):012012.
20. Kocher ET. Chirurgische Operationslehre. Jena: Fischer; 1892.
21. Motegi K. Consideration of the formation and biological significance of hypertrophic scar. J Maxillofac Surg. 1984;12:123–7.
22. Reihsner R, Balogh B, Menzel EJ. Two-dimensional elastic properties of human skin in terms of an incremental model at the in vivo configuration. Med Eng Phys. 1995;17(4):304–13.
23. Lanir Y, Fung YC. Two-dimensional mechanical properties of rabbit skin. I. Experimental system. J Biomech. 1974;7(1):29–34.
24. Lanir Y, Fung YC. Two-dimensional mechanical properties of rabbit skin. II Experimental results. J Biomech. 1974;7(2):171–82.
25. Manschot J, Wijn P, Brakkee A. The angular distribution function of elastic fibres as estimated from in vivo measurements. In: Huiskes R, van Campen DH, de Wijn JR, editors. Biomechanics, Vol. I: principles and applications. The Hague: M. Nijhoff; 1982.
26. Agache PG, Humbert P. Measuring the skin: non-invasive investigations, physiology, normal constants. Berlin: Springer; 2004. p. 435.
27. Tang J, Zeng F, Savage H, Ho PP, Alfano RR. Fluorescence spectroscopic imaging to detect changes in collagen and elastin following laser tissue welding. J Clin Laser Med Surg. 2000;18(1):3–8.
28. Mertz J, Moreaux L. Second-harmonic generation by focused excitation of in homogeneously distributed scatterers. Opt Commun. 2001;196:325–30.
29. Chen X, Nadiarynkh O, Plotnikov S, Campagnola PJ. Second harmonic generation microscopy for quantitative analysis of collagen fibrillar structure. Nat Protoc. 2012;7(4):654–69.
30. Cicchi R, Kapsokalyvas D, Troiano M, Campolmi P, Morini C, Massi D, Cannarozzo G, Lotti T, Pavone FS. In vivo non-invasive monitoring of collagen remodelling by two-photon microscopy after micro-ablative fractional laser resurfacing. J Biophotonics. 2014;7(11–12):914–25.
31. Jianxin C, et al. Multiphoton microscopy study of the morphological and quantity changes of collagen and elastic fiber components in keloid disease. J Biomed Opt. 2011;16(5):051305.
32. Riemann I, et al. In vivo multiphoton tomography of skin during wound healing and scar formation. Proc SPIE. 2007;6442:644226.
33. Paul SP, et al. A new skin tensiometer device: computational analyses to understand biodynamic excisional skin tension lines. Sci Rep. 2016;6:30117. https://doi.org/10.1038/srep30117.
34. Paul SP. The epistemology of wrinkles: from geology and anatomy to physiology. Int J Biomed. 2016;6(3):237–9.
35. Chen J, Zhuo S, Jiang X, et al. Multiphoton microscopy study of the morphological and quantity changes of collagen and elastic fiber components in keloid disease. J Biomed Opt. 2011;16(5):051305–6. https://doi.org/10.1117/1.3569617.
36. Paul SP. Are incisional and excisional skin tension lines biomechanically different? Understanding the interplay between elastin and collagen during surgical procedures. Int J Biomed. 2017;7(2):111–4.

Chapter 4
Biodynamic Excisional Skin Tension Lines: Using a New Skin Tensiometer Device and Computational Analyses to Understand Excisional Skin Biomechanics

The design brief was simple—the device developed by my team was designed to be less user-dependent, more reliable and portable for use on different bodily sites. The design and computational optimizations that we undertook are discussed here.

Our skin tensiometer needed to be bi-directional as that would enable us to study the forces needed to close cutaneous wounds and understand the differences between incisional and excisional skin lines—because as we have discussed in the previous chapter, they both have differing characteristics of elastin and collagen.

Langer, who pioneered the concept of skin tension lines, created incisional lines and noted the resultant deformation but not tension. The use of the device developed by this author's team helped to further understand skin biomechanics and map out best excisional skin tension (BEST) lines that can help plan cutaneous surgical procedures.

The author would like to acknowledge Nick Charlton, who helped design the device to the author's (often) changing specifications and Justin Matulich, who helped with computational methods including programming the software (both from the author's Design and Creative Technologies Department of the Auckland University of Technology).

4.1 Introduction

Understanding the tensile strength of wounds is critical in planning surgical techniques [1] and understanding wound healing [2]. The concept of skin tension lines is widely attributed to the studies of Langer, who used a round-tipped awl to create defects in cadaveric skin and then observed the elongation of these circular defects due to the underlying wound tension [3]. Langer perhaps never intended these lines as surgical excisional lines, even though surgeons all over the world adopted his diagrams while planning surgical procedures. Later, Borges, while studying wrinkle lines and their applications in plastic surgery, introduced the concept of skin

© Springer International Publishing AG, part of Springer Nature 2018
S. P. Paul, *Biodynamic Excisional Skin Tension Lines for Cutaneous Surgery*,
https://doi.org/10.1007/978-3-319-71495-0_4

relaxation rather than skin tension i.e. he felt skin tension rays would radiate in all directions except one and that would be the relaxed skin tension line (RSTL). He advocated planning excisions using such lines [4].

When it comes to measuring wound tension, there are generally two methods—measuring intraluminal pressure inside a hollow organ [5] or that advocated by Howe—studying the forces needed to disrupt a wound [6].

Many different tensiometers have been developed in studies to measure wound tension [2, 6] but most were cumbersome, non-portable and used clamps—the placement of which became very user-dependent. Thompson and others reported improved designs of a tensiometer to study irradiated wounds in rabbits, but images show a large non-portable device [7]. Spring-loaded sensors have also been developed to measure the force on a tensioned suture inside a closed incision and to measure the pulling force used to close the incision [8]—however, results are variable due to variability of knot-tying techniques and suture-strength.

Jacquet [9] and others have suggested when it comes to skin there is a difference with stress-strain relationships with *in vivo* and *ex vivo* measurements—if one observed the shape of the *ex vivo* test, the stress-strain curve starts with a very low slope then presents a large non-linearity at low strain, whereas in an *in vivo* test, the curve is much stiffer. This stiffness is attributed to the initial stress of the skin, also noted by Langer. Therefore, Jacquet's team designed a skin tension measuring device that relied on extensiometry testing i.e. skin was tested not only in traction, but also in compression [9]. However, this device was still not portable or user-friendly enough to be used in curved or smaller bodily sites during real-time surgery.

Our planning brief was therefore simple for this design project. Could we come up with a bi-directional skin tension measuring device that could measure inherent tension in the skin, and the force needed to close the wound i.e. one that could measure inward and outward forces while having the ease of use of a forceps? How could we achieve consistency of results while reducing the variability of readings?

4.2   Materials and Methods

The essentials of our tensiometer design and style (Fig. 4.1): The current device is designed to be used 'remotely', in other words the user is only required to operate the controls and not actually be in contact with the measuring portion of the device. This particular prototype was developed after several reviews and iterations of hand-held devices that proved to be ineffective and provided non-sensical data resulting in inaccurate readings or inconstant results.

The very first prototype we designed was based around the idea of the device operating like a pair of forceps, using the device to stretch or compress the skin, whilst using flex sensors on the arms of the device to calculate the resulting tension on the skin (Fig. 4.2). However, during the development stages several potential

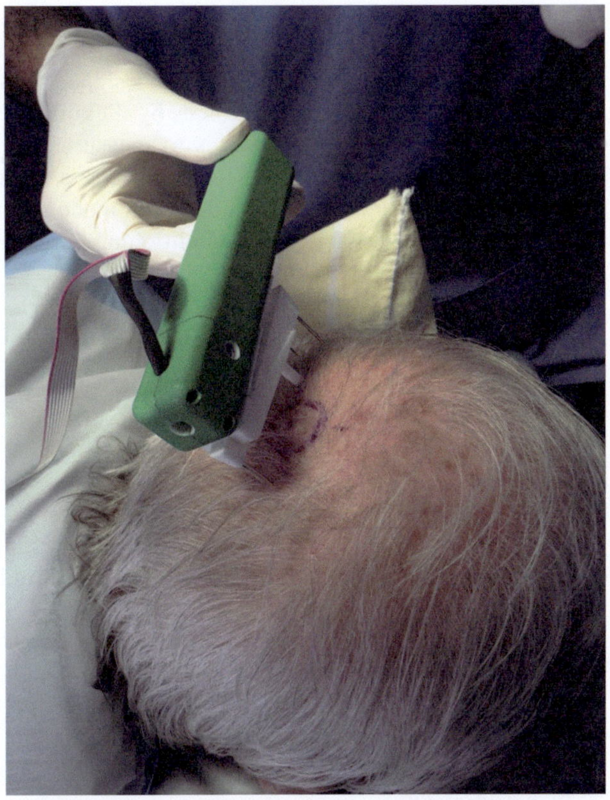

Fig. 4.1 Tensiometer being used to measure pre-tension in scalp skin prior to excision

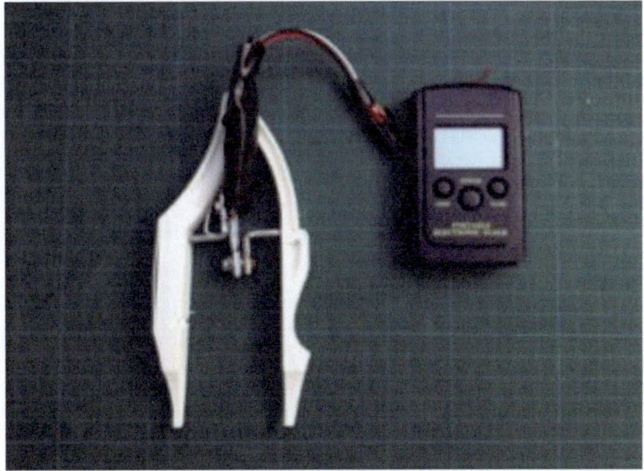

Fig. 4.2 Initial prototype was shaped like forceps, but needed modification of design

issues were discovered as to obtain consistent results the user had to apply a consistent and constant force each time a measurement was taken. Also, while using the device any instability in the user's hand caused fluctuations in the readings.

Due to the problems described above it became clear this device would need to be able to take measurements automatically without direct user support (other than operating switches). The device was also designed to be bi-directional i.e. the user can measure inward and outward forces by flicking the switch to change the direction of measurement. This allows us to measure any inherent skin tension (pretension) and understand both skin tension and relaxation lines.

Design description: The current device is made up of four main elements, a linear actuator, a force sensor, signal conditioning hardware and embedded software:

1. The linear actuator provides a consistent force that is applied to the skin to measure the resulting tension. The use of a linear actuator means if the device is securely fastened and the prongs are attached correctly then for each measurement the applied forces are consistent and repeatable. The linear actuator position is set using a varying-pulse-width waveform that is driven by a microcontroller in the control box.
2. The force sensor is a strain element force sensor with a sensing range of 0–10 Newtons (N). The reactive force applied from the skin acts via a pivoting arm on the force sensor. The force is converted to a proportional voltage potential, which is put though signal conditioning, and then converted by software into a displayable force.
3. The signal conditioning hardware is made up of an instrumentation amplifier which takes the tiny potential difference across the force sensor and amplifies it to a usable voltage. On the output stage of the amplifier is a low pass RC filter circuit with an upper cut-off frequency of 40 Hz that is used to remove high frequency noise introduced from vibrations and external interference such as the main supply hum.
4. The embedded software has three tasks, it provides the control for the linear actuator, it converts the conditioned signal voltage from the force sensor into a measurable tension, and it drives the display where the measurements are displayed.

To take a tension measurement, the software starts by taking a calibration reading, this is known as the zero tension point. The software then instructs the actuator to stretch the skin a predefined distance and the software takes another reading which is known as the final tension point. The software then instructs the actuator to return to its previous position releasing the tension on the skin. The final step is for the software to display the resulting tension which is the difference between the zero tension point and the final tension point (Tension = abs (Zero Tension Point − Final Tension Point)).

The algorithm to calculate tension is the difference between two force measurements as described above; these force measurements are derived from a digital ADC reading (0–1023) which is converted to grams using the formula (g = ADC value * 0.25). We were then able to convert this back into Newtons (N) for standardization and publication of results.

4.3   Further Technical Specifications

We used a L12-P Micro Linear Actuator with Feedback (Firgelli Technologies Inc. BC, Canada)—this device (Fig. 4.3) has an internal potentiometer that can be used to provide position feedback. However, it does not have any internal controller or limit switches.

We used a Honeywell (Honeywell Corporation, USA) Force Sensor (Fig. 4.4) with a sensing range of 0–10 N. We chose this sensor and sensing range as previous researchers have already done preliminary work to establish the range encountered in human wounds and pigskin. As we began by studying pigskin and later scalp

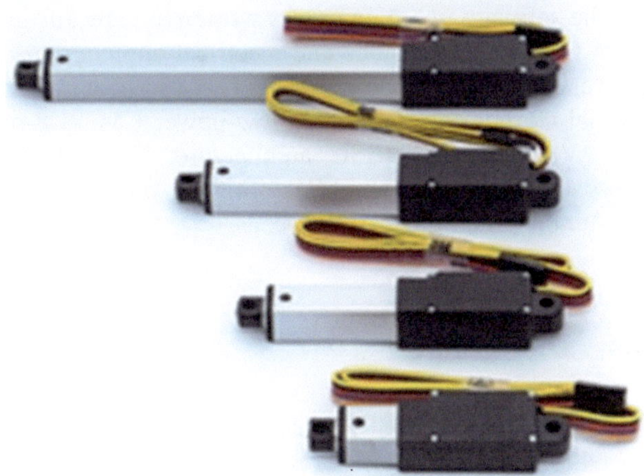

Fig. 4.3 Linear actuator with feedback

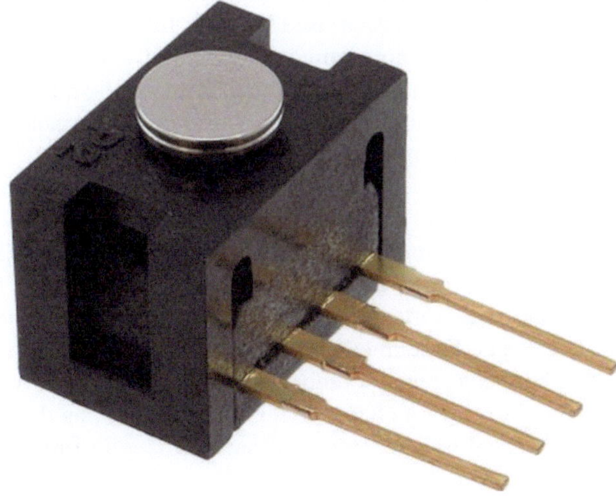

Fig. 4.4 Force sensor

skin, we looked at the kind of tension forces we would be dealing with. In human scalp wounds, it has been reported that the tension needed to approximate skin without any tension reduction suture (S) can be as high as 6.5 ± 4.6 N (Newtons) [10]. Other researchers who tested human skin over the trunk concluded the maximal force varied from 0.5 N for small wounds (30 * 5 mm) to 1.5 N for medium-sized wounds (30 * 15 mm), to a peak force of 3.2 N for large (46 * 13 mm) wounds [11]. Authors studying pigskin by creating massive elliptical defects (8 cm * 5 cm) reported the mean force needed to close non-undermined surgical wounds was 15.7 N compared with 11.5 N for undermined wounds [12]. Given we set out to investigate skin tension lines after excisional surgery for skin cancer, we determined a range of 0–10 N was adequate for our purposes. In our testing on scalp wounds, we found a range of tension measurements from 0.5 to 4.6 N.

The software in our case, was written in C by Justin Matulich, a member of our team from the electronics and electrical engineering department at the Auckland University of Technology (AUT). The microcontroller used was the ATMEGA32 (Atmel Corporation, USA)—a low-power CMOS 8-bit microcontroller based on the AVR enhanced RISC architecture. The ATmega32 achieves throughputs approaching 1 MIPS per MHz allowing our system designer to optimize power consumption and processing speeds.

4.4   Discussion

We developed an initial prototype that was tested on pigskin (Fig. 4.5) and optimised to achieve consistent results before the final design with autoclave-able tips for human skin was made (Fig. 4.1). Domesticated pigs are the most common animal model for skin testing as they have skin that is similar to human skin, and Yorkshire pigs have been used to study full-thickness skin wounds because unlike other pigs, they do not change weight rapidly if calorie-restricted [13]. In pigs, tension lines run oblique to vertebrae in the cephalic area, perpendicular to vertebrae in the middle torso, and parallel to vertebrae in the caudal area, and this finding has been consistent across porcine species' studies [14].

In pigskin we used our device to test wound tension for primary elliptical surgical closures and to compare and contrast different cutaneous flap techniques, the results of which are the basis of different chapters in this book. On the scalp, the device allowed us a great understanding of the biodynamics of Langer's, Kraissl's, and Borges's lines and determination of the best methods of closing scalp defects. Fundamentally we were able to determine the biomechanical differences between 'tension' and 'relaxation' skin lines. Again, these findings will be detailed in relevant chapters, region by region, as the objective here is to present our new innovative tensiometer that was a major improvement on previous devices of this nature.

The device we used for measuring BEST lines has been previously described and detailed in another article [15]. In our final design, we incorporated a bracing bar

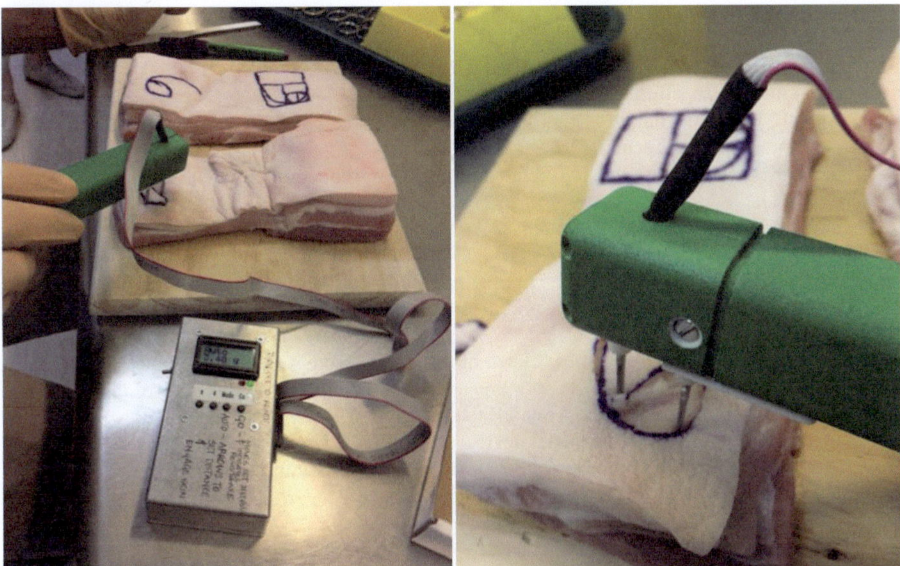

Fig. 4.5 Tensiometer being used to compare different flap designs on pigskin

that steadies the device and negates any operational hand tremors. However, it does take some understanding and practice to use the device and achieve completely reliable results. In our case, the lead author has now been able to use the device in different settings and achieve consistent results and make observations that can be extrapolated in various clinical settings. The system, while intended as a research tool and not as a commercial device was relatively portable and had the ability to measure skin tension for any zone and body site—which our team believed was a major advance over previous devices [15].

In this treatise, the author will specifically describe BEST lines in different anatomical locations and these will be presented in further chapters of this book.

References

1. Milch RA. Tensile strength of surgical wounds. J Surg Res. 1965;5:377.
2. Sandbloom P, Peterson P, Musen A. Determination of the tensile strength of the healing wound as a clinical test. Acta Chir Scand. 1953;105:552.
3. Langer K. On the anatomy and physiology of the skin, The Imperial Academy of Science, Vienna. Reprinted in (1978): Br J Plast Surg. 1861;17(31):93–106.
4. Borges AF. Relaxed skin tension lines (RSTL) versus other skin lines. Plast Reconstr Surg. 1984;73(1):144–50.
5. Howes EL, Sooy J, Harvey SC. Healing of wounds as determined by their tensile strength. JAMA. 1929;92:42.
6. Botsford TW. The tensile strength of sutured skin wounds during healing. Surg Gynecol Obstet. 1941;72:690.

7. Thompson LW, Zook EG, Hugo NE. A tensiometer to measure wound tensile strength in situ. J Surg Res. 1969;9(9):543–6.
8. Horeman T, Meijer E-J, Harlaar JJ, Lange JF, van den Dobbelsteen JJ, Dankelman J. Force sensing in surgical sutures. PLoS One. 2013;8(12):e84466.
9. Jacquet E, Josse G, Khatyr F, Garcin CA. new experimental method for measuring skin's natural tension. Skin Res Technol. 2008;14:1–7.
10. Hwang K, et al. Skin tension related to tension reduction sutures. J Craniofac Surg. 2015;26(1):e48.
11. Capek L, Jacquet E, et al. The analysis of forces needed for the suturing of elliptical skin wounds. Med Biol Eng Comput. 2012;50:193–8.
12. Tønseth KA, Hokland BM. Evaluation of microcirculation and wound-closing tension after undermining the skin: a study in a porcine model using laser Doppler perfusion imaging. Eur J Plast Surg. 2004;27:295–7.
13. Yabuki A. Skin morphology of the clawn miniature pig. Exp Anim. 2007;56:369–73.
14. Kwak M, Son D, et al. Static Langer's line and wound contraction rates according to anatomical regions in a porcine model. Wound Repair Regen. 2014;22:678–82.
15. Paul SP, et al. A new skin tensiometer device: computational analyses to understand biodynamic excisional skin tension lines. Sci Rep. 2016;6(30117). https://doi.org/10.1038/srep30117.

Chapter 5
Biodynamic Excisional Skin Tension (BEST) Lines for Scalp Reconstruction After Skin Cancer Surgery

5.1 Scalp Anatomy

The five layers of the scalp are often remembered by the mnemonic SCALP (Skin; Connective Tissue; Aponeurosis; Loose Areolar Tissue; Pericranium) [1]. When it comes to skin thickness, scalp skin is thicker than most body sites with skin thickness ranging from 3 mm (vertex) to 8 mm (occiput) [2]. The scalp has a large concentration of sebaceous glands, and this not only makes scalp skin oily, but leads to the relatively common occurrence of trichilemmal/sebaceous cysts [1]. The connective tissue is bound by fibrous septae into which blood vessels retract when we incise the scalp (or when the scalp is lacerated by injury). Authors have described two techniques to stem bleeding on the scalp (1) The surgeon or assistant presses firmly down on the underlying skull with his fingers, thus compressing vessels, or (2) Artery forceps can be placed on the aponeurotic layer and scalp flaps are turned over thereby compressing the bleeding blood vessels [2]. However, this abundance of blood vessels on the scalp means that flaps with narrow pedicles have a higher survival rate here than on anywhere else on the body. This must be tempered by the fact that the scalp is not supplied by musculocutaneous perforators. It is therefore very important to not transect larger blood vessels in the periphery of the scalp, as this will result in a loss of blood supply over scalp skin.

One of the other interesting and lesser known aspects of scalp vascularity is the differences between hair-bearing and non-hair-bearing areas. It is known that hair follicles are situated in the upper part of the subcutis and the hair follicles are nourished by a subcutaneous plexus [3]. Studies have been done using local ^{133}Xe clearance method, a method in which the tracer was injected intracutaneously to avoid interference from injection trauma in the subcutaneous tissue allowing the researcher to focus on the upper subcutaneous tissue [3]. A similar study using local ^{133}Xe clearance method was also done previously in patients with alopecia areata [4]. More recently, Doppler flow and thermography studies also confirmed that areas of scalp devoid of hair have a reduced blood flow [5]. These studies reveal that in both

© Springer International Publishing AG, part of Springer Nature 2018
S. P. Paul, *Biodynamic Excisional Skin Tension Lines for Cutaneous Surgery*,
https://doi.org/10.1007/978-3-319-71495-0_5

male pattern baldness and alopecia areata, the finding is that cutaneous and subcutaneous blood flow is reduced in bald scalp areas—and this has implications during surgery for both skin cancer and hair transplantation.

The galea aponeurotica derives its name from Roman soldiers' helmets (Latin galea = helmet). The significance of the galeal layer was noted by Harvey Cushing, during his time as a military surgeon when he emphasized the significance of closing the galea [6]. The galea varies in thickness from 1 to 2 mm and is better developed in some individuals [7]. It must be considered part of the occipitofrontalis muscle as it drapes over the vertex of the skull between the frontal and occipital bellies of this muscle. The occipital belly may be able to be contracted in some individuals, but usually only anchors the aponeurosis. In contrast, the contraction of the frontal belly or frontalis elevates the eyebrows and is the cause for the horizontal creases we note on foreheads [7].

The subgaleal space or the loose areolar tissue lends itself to easy surgical dissection. Scalp skin can be easily peeled away when one is this surgical plane, an anatomical fact well known to Native Americans during the process of "scalping". One of the practical implications of this loose areolar tissue during surgery is that if a surgeon confines surgical dissection to the subgaleal plane during cutaneous surgery, the blood supply to the skin flaps is not compromised in any way. Because of this unique anatomy, undermining is not useful on the scalp as it is in other parts of the body. Seery after undertaking a review of over 3000 scalp operations concluded, "I have found that in very lax scalps, it is possible to remove 5 cm widths at the midsagittal ellipse level and yet easily close the wound without any undermining. Conversely, in tight scalps, removing 5 cm and achieving closure is impossible regardless of the extent of undermining." This led to the conclusion that the more important factor, by far, in determining the extent of tissue amenable to excision is not the extent of undermining, but the degree of laxity. It was also concluded that "the extent of undermining and tissue amenable to removal are not linearly related" [7]. Where the galea is poorly developed in individuals, the pericranium makes a good substitute [8]. This knowledge is also useful during surgery, with authors describing techniques of suturing the galea to pericranium to reduce tension vector forces in scalp tissues, a method that results in a 39 mm reduction with a 13% stretch-back or a theoretical 34 mm gain [8].

Ultimately, from a surgical anatomy point of view the scalp has different properties in different regions. We have just discussed that the scalp has five layers. But this is only true of the subgaleal space. This five-layered scalp is where scalp flaps can be easily mobilized with minimal dissection or bleeding. The rest of the scalp has three layers: skin, subcutaneous tissues, and deep fascia (Fig. 5.1)—the latter is the same fascia that continues over the trapezius and sternomastoid muscles.

Given the surgical anatomy of the scalp has some unique considerations, Olson and Hamilton list the following points as the mainstays to understanding scalp reconstruction [9]: The loss of hair-bearing skin poses unique challenges in reconstruction especially given that we know that non-hair bearing tissues have different vascularity. Further, the scalp due to the galea aponeurosis layer is less elastic than other areas of the head and neck, making reconstruction challenging.

Fig. 5.1 Illustration of the anatomical areas where the scalp has three and five layers

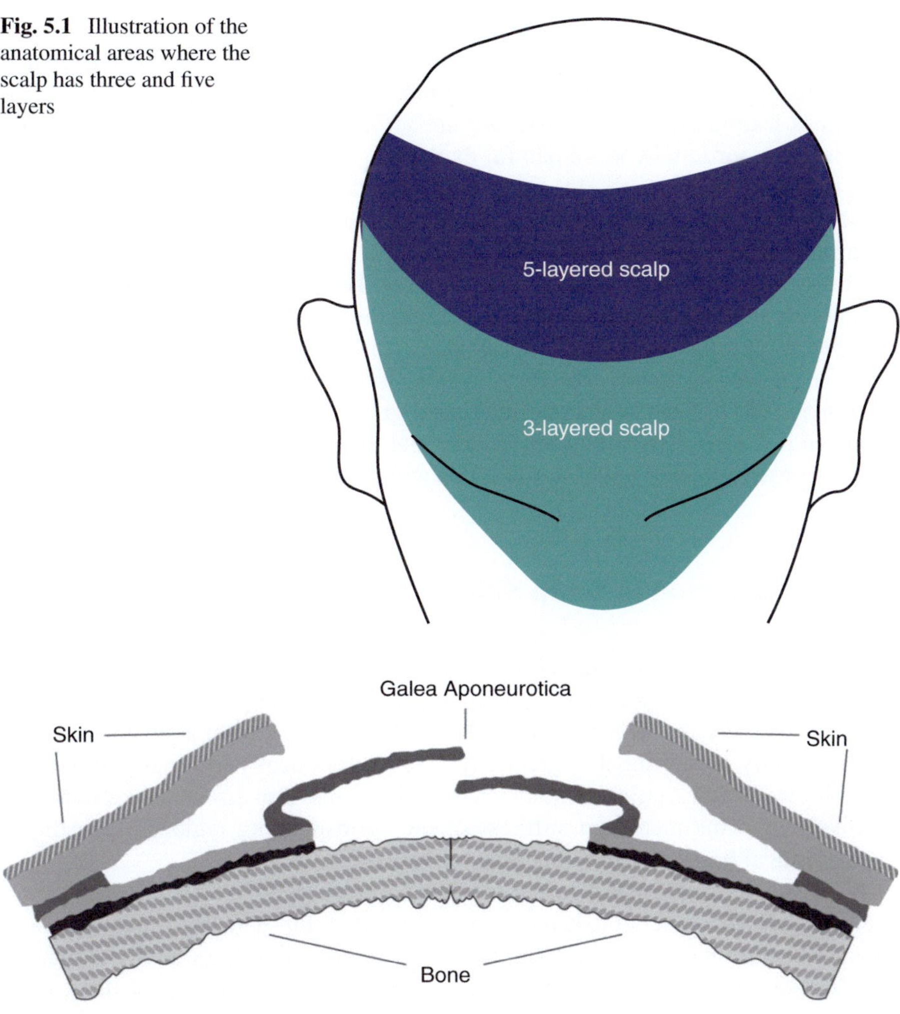

Fig. 5.2 Galeal flap that can be used to cover bare bone defects

Because the galea makes the scalp relatively inelastic, closing the wound under excessive tension can lead to necrosis of skin and the patient can end up with a barebone defect that will not take a skin graft. Authors have described flaps (Fig. 5.2) raised from the galea that can cover bare-bone defects and take skin grafts as an alternative to flap closures [10].

And, we now know that in non-bald scalps each scalp layer changes with aging and the most noticeable changes are in the layers that contain hair [11]. We also know that the condition of the galea is influenced by aging in advanced baldness and that all skin layers except the galea exhibit definite thinning. In contrast, in bald subjects early male pattern loss of hair is accompanied by no changes in scalp thickness [11].

We know that skin stretch attenuates blood vessels and decreases tissue perfusion. As the tension increases or the skin is stretched beyond its elastic limit, tension will ultimately exceed the critical closing pressure of the blood vessels and perfusion stops leading to skin necrosis. We already know that closing a wound under tension is proportionally more painful than when skin is closed under less tension. This is because nerves are elongated and a similar stretch of lymphatics leads to tissue edema. The elastic limit for skin elastin is generally about 10% and that for collagen is 100%. What this means is, even a 10% elongation of skin over its resting length ends up causing a rupture of elastin fibres. The problem is, even if the tension is removed, this impairment is irreversible and this impaired elastin is now no longer able to return to its normal resting state. This permanent irremediable adverse event is known as stretch atrophy [7]. Defects can be less than a centimetre or encompass most of the scalp, and may need grafts flaps or multiple techniques—therefore it is especially important to orientate the initial lines of closure properly under least tension, and understanding this will be the focus of this chapter.

5.2   Introduction to Scalp Skin Dynamics

The most important initial step in planning an elliptical excision is determining the proper anatomical orientation of the ellipse [12]. It is well known in the practice of cutaneous surgery that when it comes to scar formation, greater skin stress or tension is directly proportional to greater (and less cosmetically ideal) scar formation [13]. Several studies on skin biomechanics show that skin stress values correlate positively with the measured stiffness of the corresponding region, suggesting a biomechanical basis for exuberant scar formation [14].

Karl Langer, as discussed earlier, conducted pioneering studies into skin cleavage lines that were first published in 1861. He created skin-defects in cadavers using a round-tipped awl, and then noted the direction in which these clefts elongated [15]. Langer perhaps never intended these lines as surgical excisional lines, even though surgeons all over the world began adopting his diagrams even for scalp surgery. Langer did note that the causes for skin tension were two-fold—physiological (such as displacement due to fat) or pathological (due to an underlying mass or tumour), and contour lines caused by the movement of joints [15]. These factors often lead to errors in ellipse placement—as underlying joint movement or patient posture on the operating table may lead to altered tension on the skin.

Nearly a century after Langer, in 1941, HT Cox from Manchester, used a marlin-spike and recreated Langer's experiment [16]. Cornelius Kraissl, from New York, took photographs of people when muscles of facial expression were contracted, and then a composite sketch was drawn of his "wrinkle lines". He found quite a bit of individual variation on the face and scalp due to differences in contour or muscle development [17]. Kraissl felt his wrinkle lines in general ran perpendicular to muscle-fibre direction. Notably, on the scalp Kraissl's lines differ markedly from Langer's lines, yet both have been considered appropriate for use in surgical excisions. Alberto Borges was of the view that tension is present in all directions except one, and he coined the term relaxed skin tension lines (RSTL) which became his preferred direction for wound closures on the face [18].

Knowledge of relaxed skin tension lines is essential to anyone that practices cutaneous surgery. Such investigation and decision-making using applied surgical anatomy is considered central to plastic surgical practice [19]. But can such a technique of merely pinching skin, as advocated by Borges [18] be scientifically robust and accurate on an area like the scalp? While skin is anisotropic, it is especially more orthotropic close to bone i.e. have directional symmetry and hence the importance of determining the preferential direction for wound closure after excision of skin cancers on the scalp. The author used a previously developed and described bi-directional skin tension-measuring device to measure best excisional skin tension (BEST) lines at different sites [20]. BEST lines are, as the name indicates the best lines of closure for *excisional* wounds.

Fundamentally, this study set out to study the biomechanical differences between 'tension' and 'relaxation' skin lines and to map out the best excisional skin tension (BEST) lines of the scalp i.e. the preferred direction to orientate the wound closure after excisional surgery under the least possible tension.

5.3   Materials and Methods

The tensiometer that was used in this study to determine biodynamic excisional skin tension (BEST) lines has already been the subject of another paper, and the mechanism discussed in detail [20]. It consists of four main elements, a linear actuator, a force sensor, signal conditioning hardware and embedded software. This device is bi-directional i.e. the user can measure inward and outward forces by flicking the switch to change the direction of measurement. This allows us to measure any inherent skin tension (pre-tension) to help understand both skin tension and relaxation lines (Fig. 5.3).

A formal study was undertaken in patients, after obtaining ethics committee approvals—New Zealand: Health and Disability Ethics Committee (HDEC Reference No. 15/CEN/113); Australia: University of Queensland Institutional Human Ethics (Approval No. 2015001550). This study was carried out in accordance with the recommendations of the ethics committees listed above, with written informed consent from all subjects. All subjects gave written informed consent in accordance with the Declaration of Helsinki.

In our tensiometer, measurements of tension are made when the software takes a calibration reading—the zero-tension point. The linear actuator then stretches the skin, as if pulling the wound closed and another reading is taken—the final-tension point. The software is programmed to display the skin tension reading i.e. the difference between the zero-tension point and the final-tension point.

Once the machine was tested and calibrated as per previously published testing protocols [20], the author set out to use the device to measure tension in different directions on the scalp—coronal, sagittal and oblique (Fig. 5.4). Lesions were marked out in a circular fashion and converted to elliptical closures, once the

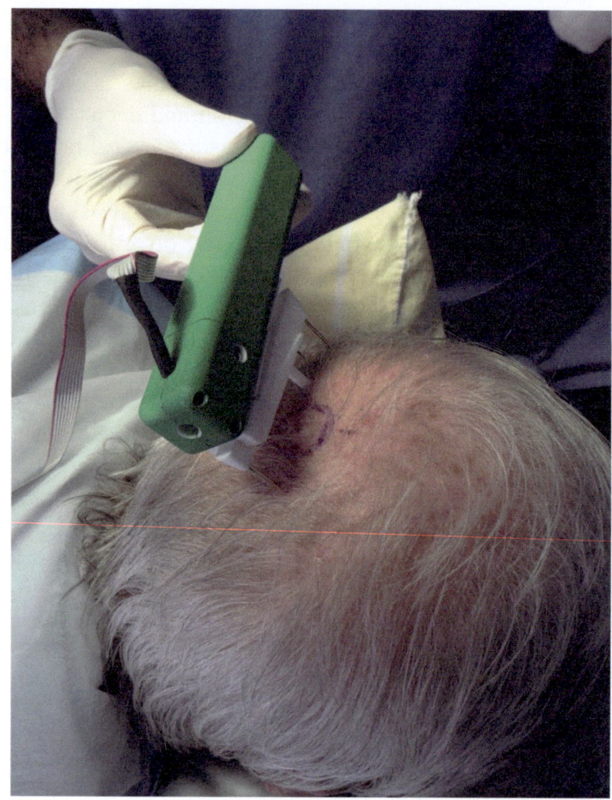

Fig. 5.3 Measuring tension using tensiometer (in this figure any inherent pre-tension)

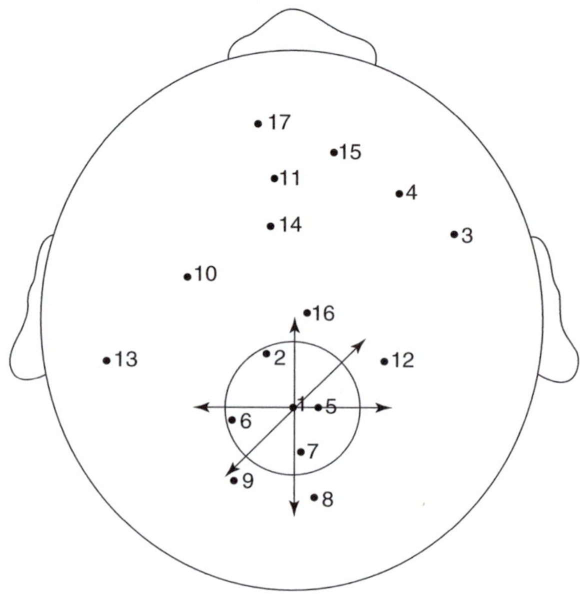

Fig. 5.4 Tension measurements in different directions

preferential line of closure i.e. BEST line was established. Even when the lesion was too large to close primarily and a cutaneous flap was needed, the final closure was orientated after determining the best line of closure.

Skin tensions were measured for 17 different scalp wounds created after excision of skin cancers. Any pre-tension i.e. preferential direction prior to creation of the defect was noted. There was considerable individual variation in skin tension and all readings were recorded. Patients that had lesions on old radiotherapy or cryotherapy scars were not included in this study.

Once measurements were completed, a detailed statistical analysis of our findings was undertaken by our statistics department, which has special expertise in applied mathematics for biomechanical experiments.

5.4 Results

Depending on the size and site of the wounds on the scalp, "tension fields" varied from 0.2 to 6 N (Table 5.1). The site of each lesion on the scalp has been depicted in the illustration (Fig. 5.4). Anatomically, lesions at the vertex and occiput of the scalp had the most tension, even when lesion size was accounted for; directionally, coronal closures had the *least* tension, and oblique closures had the *greatest* tension. Interestingly, when the wound diameter was under 0.7 cm, coronal and sagittal direction closures had similar tension. Most wounds over 2 cm had some outward "pre-tension"—inherent

Table 5.1 Force measured in N for coronal, sagittal and oblique closures of circular wounds scalp

No.	Outward pre-tension	Coronal (transverse) force (N)/tension	Galeal scoring	Oblique force (N)/tension	Sagittal (vertical) force (N)/tension	Defect size (cm)
1	0.4	4.6	4.0 (13%)	6.0	4.9	3
2	0.0	3.2	3.8	3.5	3	
3	0.1	3.0		3.2	3.0	4
4	0.2	2.4		2.6	2.4	2
5	0.4	1.8		2.8	2.1	4
6	0.1	1.1		1.4	1.1	2.5
7	0.2	3.2	2.9 (9.3%)	4.2	3.6	3
8	0.0	1.9		3.2	2.9	2.5
9	0.3	3.2		4.2	3.6	2
10	0.4	4.0	3.5 (12.5%)	5.0	4.6	2.5
11	0.6	3.2		4.9	3.7	2
12	0.6	3.7	3.3 (10.8%)	4.7	3.9	4
13	0.5	3.0		4.0	3.6	3
14	0.0	0.7		1.0	0.7	0.7
15	0.0	0.7		0.9	0.7	0.6
16	0.0	0.4		0.5	0.4	0.4
17	0.0	0.9		0.2	0.9	0.7

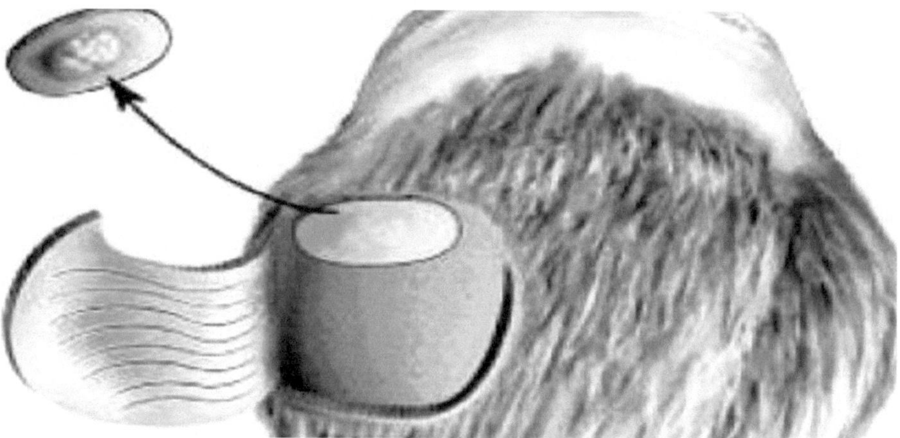

Fig. 5.5 Galeal scoring to reduce wound tension

outward pull prior to excision, but once the lesion was excised and the defect was created, the tension was least in the coronal direction. We can now understand why surgeons sometimes mistakenly orient excisions in either the vertical or oblique planes, as pinching scalp skin can give an erroneous finding, especially when there are other scars present or the patient's head is positioned on a pillow. Under 0.7 cm, there was no "pretension" noted. In four cases, as the wounds were very large, the galea (aponeurosis) layer was scored (also in a coronal fashion) to reduce wound tension and such 'galeal scoring' reduces wound tension by 9–13% (Fig. 5.5).

The results presented here, show clearly that the tension is lowest in the coronal direction, and therefore the best excisional skin tension lines (BEST) on the scalp run in a coronal direction i.e. transverse left-to-right direction (Fig. 5.2). The overall direction of RSTL lines on the scalp are not dissimilar to BEST lines, although they are not identical lines. As noted, further reduction in tension can be achieved by scoring the scalp's aponeurosis layer (this is also done in a coronal fashion), when needed. The galea can also be utilized to cover bare bone defects that will not take a skin graft. Given the unique galeal anatomy, a galea-only flap can be raised that can be stretched over to cover a bare bone defect and a skin graft overlaid on the galeal flap (Fig. 5.2).

Some wounds exhibited an inherent outward force (wound gape) but this did not have a bearing on wound closures as in all cases tension was least in the coronal (transverse) direction of the scalp.

Discussions were undertaken with our statistics and mathematical sciences department to determine the best methodology to use for analysis. In this case, two-sided paired t-tests were applied. The team compared wound tension prior to closure in the coronal, sagittal and oblique planes. The coronal tension was noted to be significantly different (less) when compared with both the sagittal and oblique skin tension measurements (two-sided paired t-test, unequal variances; $p = 0.00075$ and 0.000013 respectively). Irrespective of the location on the scalp, wound closures in coronal fashion had the least tension and hence we can expect best outcomes.

5.5 Discussion

The scalp has unique dynamics due to the presence of the aponeurosis layer, the galea, and the attachments of the occipitofrontalis muscle. Langer's lines (Fig. 5.6 illustrates Langer's lines in green colour) have long been considered static, although researchers have suggested that these lines are direction-dependent and dynamic—with changes occurring due to movement of joints or bodily units. On the scalp, Borges lines run coronally (transversely). Figure 5.6 shows the comparison (and contrast) between Langer's, Kraissl's and Borges's lines on the scalp—Langer's lines are illustrated in green, while Borges's lines are blue, and Kraissl's lines are shown in red.

Borges' method of pinching skin, is not always reliable, especially when there is pre-existing scarring or radiotherapy. We report a patient in whom ellipses had been marked by pinching skin, but he ended up with skin grafts on his scalp as the wounds could not be closed primarily, as illustrated in the (Fig. 5.7). In our case, a coronal ellipse achieved closure for a defect of similar dimension (this was determined from reviewing the previous operation notes and histology samples).

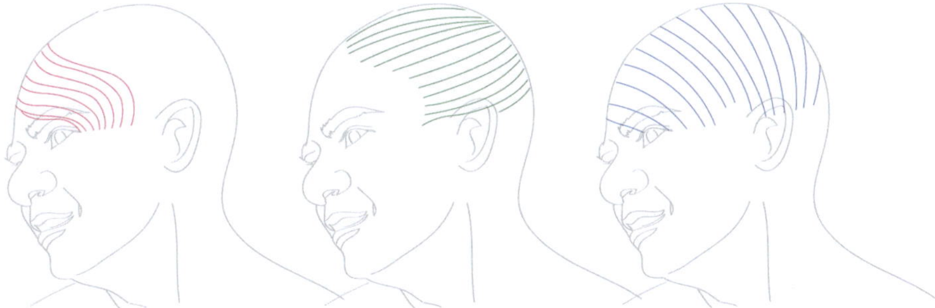

Fig. 5.6 Different skin lines illustrated Langer (green) Kraissl (red) Borges (blue)

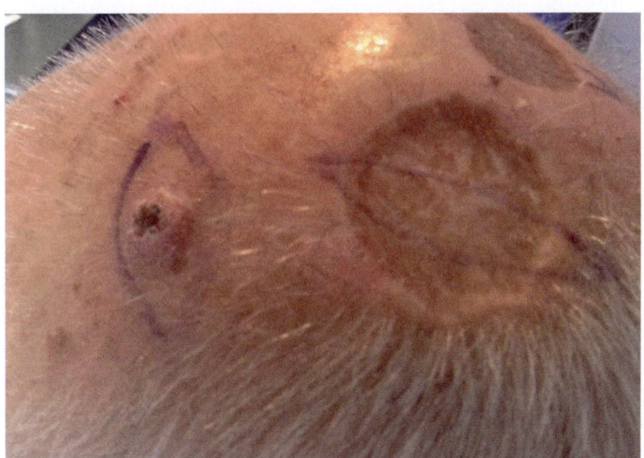

Fig. 5.7 Ellipses marked inaccurately can lead to unnecessary skin grafts

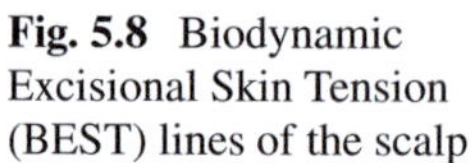

Fig. 5.8 Biodynamic Excisional Skin Tension (BEST) lines of the scalp

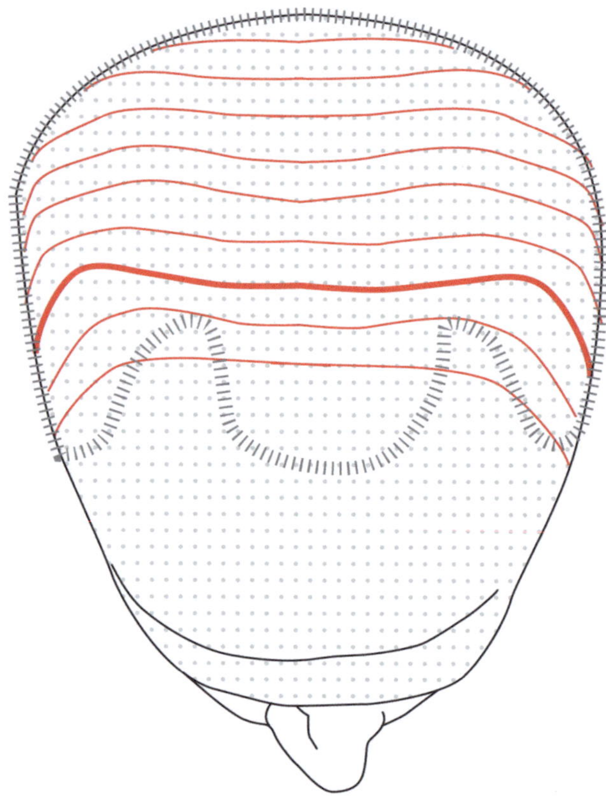

In fact, this patient (Fig. 5.7) was placed on the author's operating list for a skin graft because the scalp was deemed too tight for primary closure given his two previous failed attempts (when the ellipse had been marked using Langer's lines as a guide as illustrated in Fig. 5.7). Our study may also explain why Langer's lines on the scalp run vertically, as Langer's experiment was a study of cleavage lines and not excisional lines—again confirming the author's view that excisional and incisional lines are indeed biomechanically different across the body.

The findings in this study show that closing tension is least when an ellipse is planned in a coronal fashion (transverse or left-to-right direction) on the scalp, and therefore, as far as the scalp is concerned the best excisional skin tension (BEST) lines are coronal (Fig. 5.8). We found that the convex nature of the scalp does not seem to matter because of the lack of attachment of the underlying galeal aponeurosis (except in the frontal and occipital regions), and this may be why the BEST lines on the scalp are coronal. And, when the diameter of the defect is under 7 mm, direction does not seem to matter much as the inherent tension is minimal.

Most surgeons excise a lesion, thereby creating a defect, and physically assess the best direction of closure by pinching skin or attempting to draw wound edges together. Some practitioners mark the direction of an ellipse beforehand—based on their assessment of the laxity of the skin. The information obtained in this study regarding best excisional skin tension (BEST) lines for scalp closures is valuable because it gives the surgeon a general rule to follow. In Australia and New Zealand, scalp skin cancers are exceptionally common due to high UV damage—especially on patients with bald heads, and many of these lesions are often dealt with in primary care. Given there was a clear reduction in wound tension when coronal closures are performed, this directional guidance (Fig. 5.8 indicates BEST lines on the scalp) will also be of great help to those planning elliptical excisions of skin cancers in an office procedure-room setting.

The author has previously published this research into scalp skin tension and biodynamics, based on experiments conducted to specifically study BEST lines of the scalp—research that revisited the concepts behind Langer's Lines, and confirmed the concepts behind BEST Lines [21]. These findings can be summarized thus [21]:

1. Biodynamic Excisional Skin Tension (BEST) lines on the scalp run coronally (transversely) and this should be the preferred orientation of wound closures on the scalp.
2. For further reduction in tension to the order of approximately one-tenths, galeal scoring can be useful.
3. For very small defects such as those that would occur after traumatic lacerations, directional forces seem equivalent in all directions

References

1. Ellis H, Mahadevan V. The surgical anatomy of the scalp. Surgery. 2013;32:S1.
2. Matloub H, Molnar J. Anatomy of the scalp. In: Stough D, Haber R, editors. Hair replacement. St. Louis: Mosby; 1996. p. 20.
3. Klemp P, Lindskov R, Staberg B. Subcutaneous blood flow in alopecia areata. Clin Exp Dermatol. 1984;9(2):181–5.
4. Beurey J, Weber M, Bertrand A, Robert J, Mabille H. Mesure du debit vasculaire des plaques peladiques au moyen du xenon 123. Bull Soc Fr Dermatol Syphiligr. 1972;79:176–9.
5. Toshitani S, Nakayama J, Yahata T, Yasuda M, Urabe H. A new apparatus for hair regrowth in male-pattern baldness. J Dermatol. 1990;17(4):240–6.
6. Cushing H. Surgery of the head. In: Keen WW, editor. Surgery: its principles and practice, vol. 3. Philadelphia: WB Saunders; 1908. p. 17–276.
7. Seery GE. Surgical anatomy of the scalp. Dermatol Surg. 2002;28(7):581–7.
8. Seery GE. Galea fixation. Dermatol Surg. 2001;27:931–6.
9. Olson M, Hamilton GS. Scalp and forehead defects in the post-Mohs surgery patient. Facial Plast Surg Clin North Am. 2017;25(3):365–75.
10. Prera E, Pfeiffer J. Galea-aponeurotic flap for the repair of large scalp defects extending to bone. Auris Nasus Larynx. 2015;42:156–9.
11. Hori H, Moretti G, Rebora A, Crovato F. The thickness of human scalp: normal and bald. J Invest Dermatol. 1972;58(6):396–9.
12. Leshin B, Dunlavey E. The simple excision. Dermatol Clin. 1998;16(1):49–64. https://doi.org/10.1016/S0733-8635(05)70486-1.

13. Meyer M, McGrouther DA. A study relating wound tension to scar morphology in the pre-sternal scar using Langers technique. Br J Plast Surg. 1991;44:291–4. https://doi.org/10.1016/0007-1226(91)90074-T.
14. Wong VW, Levi K, Akaishi S, Schultz G, Dauskardt RH. Scar zones: region-specific differences in skin tension may determine incisional scar formation. Plast Reconstr Surg. 2012;129(6):1272–6. https://doi.org/10.1097/PRS.0b013e31824eca79.
15. Langer K. On the anatomy and physiology of the skin (1861), The Imperial Academy of Science, Vienna. Reprinted in: Br J Plast Surg. 1978;17(31):93–106.
16. Cox HT. The cleavage lines of the skin. Br J Surg. 1941;29:234–40.
17. Kraissl CJ. The selection of appropriate lines for elective surgical incisions. Plast Reconstr Surg. 1951;8(1):1–28.
18. Borges AF, Alexander JE. Relaxed skin tension lines, z-plasties on scars, and fusiform excision of lesions. Br J Plast Surg. 1962;15:242–54. https://doi.org/10.1016/S0007-1226(62)80038-1.
19. Gillespie RH, Banwell RS, Hormbrey EL, Inglefield CJ, Roberts AHN. A new model for assessment in plastic surgery: knowledge of relaxed skin tension lines. Br J Plast Surg. 2000;53(3):243–4. https://doi.org/10.1054/bjps.1999.3265.
20. Paul SP, Matulich J, Charlton NA. New skin tensiometer device: computational analyses to understand biodynamic excisional skin tension lines. Sci Rep. 2016;6:30117. https://doi.org/10.1038/srep30117.
21. Paul SP. Revisiting Langer's lines, introducing BEST lines, and studying the biomechanics of scalp skin. Spectr Dermatol. 2017;2:8–11.

Chapter 6
Golden Spirals and Scalp Whorls:
Nature's Patterns and the Designing
of a New Scalp Flap

6.1 Studying Nature's Own Design

One of my roles is as an Adjunct Professor in the Department of Design and Creative Technology. My main interest, other than in integrating medicine and engineering design is in fostering creativity and disruptive innovation.

The following experiment documents what began as an exercise in curiosity—logarithmic spiral designs abound in nature—in galaxies, flowers, even pinecones, and on human scalps as whorls. Why are humans the only primates to have whorls on the scalp? Is the formation of scalp whorls mechanical or genetic? A mechanical theory has long been postulated—the mechanical theory suggests that hair whorl patterning is determined by the tension on the epidermis during rapid expansion of the cranium while the hair follicle is growing downwards—however, this has never before, to the author's knowledge, been experimentally proven conclusively. This experiment was essentially conducted to understand skin dynamics and especially the changes that occur in tissue when confronted by expansive forces.

Logarithmic spirals such as golden spirals (with a growth factor of $\phi = 1.6180339887$, the golden ratio) are ubiquitous in nature and are seen in arrangements of leaves, seeds, pinecones and many different arrangements in nature [1]. Such spiral patterns are frequently observed and utilized in a variety of phenomena including galaxies, biological organisms, as well as turbulent flows [2]. Many have attributed mysticism to the presence of origins—the golden ratio was called τ (tau), the symbol of life, and was also known to ancient Egyptians (the ankh) and Hindus [3]. One of the viewpoints for the occurrence in plants was inherently protoplasmic i.e. "spirals" exist in nature through constitutional rather than external mechanical influences [4]. However, a team noted that metallic nanoparticles could be made to arrange themselves with floral spiral design and commented that the shape of spirals depended on size of particles, thickness of shell and rate of cooling [5]. Others have stimulated spiral wave forms in neuronal circuits of the human body [6]. While Fibonacci spirals are everywhere in nature, and indeed common in art and

© Springer International Publishing AG, part of Springer Nature 2018
S. P. Paul, *Biodynamic Excisional Skin Tension Lines for Cutaneous Surgery*,
https://doi.org/10.1007/978-3-319-71495-0_6

architecture—in a laboratory setting, spontaneous assembly of such patterns has rarely been realized in mechanical tests, and never previously on skin [6]. Some researchers demonstrated Fibonacci spiral patterns could be reproduced through stress manipulation on the metal-core based shell microstructures and commented on the possible role of mechanical stress in influencing these spiral patterns [7]. And, in a study of rocks and tectonic plates, researchers noted spiral patterns of cracks—where the cracking arises not from twisting forces but from a progressing stress front [8].

As an animal biologist and skin cancer academic, the author's fascination has been with the fact that humans are the only animals to have scalp whorls on the top of their heads that follow spiral patterns seen in nature. Others have noted that of all mammals, only humans have hair whorls on the vertex of the scalp, and that each human individual *must* have a hair whorl [9]. Animals like horses do have whorls on the body or faces, but not on the top of their heads—and this is *not* universal in all horses—however, such patterns demonstrate less variability, and show more Mendelian forms of inheritance than those seen in humans [10]. In keeping with such genetic theories, the number of whorls on a horse's face and the direction of such patterns are used to gauge equine temperament such as calmness, enthusiasm or wariness [11]. Notably, other primates like chimpanzees, that are evolutionarily closer to humans, do not have whorls [12]. In this experiment, we attempted to recreate skin whorls by causing shearing forces due to *rapid* skin expansion, along a progressing front.

6.2   Materials and Methods

6.2.1   The Medium

The author spent a whole year in testing and studying the properties of pigskin, and its suitability as an equivalent and comparable testing medium to human skin, before formally testing the mechanical theory of spiral formations in organic tissue. This involved considerable time taken to perfect the technique of creating rapid dermo-epidermal shear by inflating a saline expander rapidly.

Pigskin has been noted to be the closest medium to human skin in several studies—Herron noted that pigs were the ideal dermatological models in skin surgery, wound healing, burns and skin therapies such as lasers [12]. Schmook and others compared human and animal skin and concluded that "in agreement with published data, pigskin appeared as the most suitable model for human skin: the fluxes through the skin and concentrations in the skin were of the same order of magnitude for both tissues" [13].

Before one can study skin biodynamics or surgical closure techniques, one needs a good understanding of the directions of skin tension lines of normal skin. Karl Langer (1819–1887), as we have discussed, was one of the earliest people to undertake such studies, when he undertook experiments to study physical and mechanical properties of human skin [14] in cadavers by making small circular incisions on skin—and then noting the directions they were distorted in—these 'skin tension lines' he termed "cleavage lines" [15]. Since Langer's original study, many other variations of skin tension lines have been mapped out—and people have noted that in certain parts of the face, Langer's lines deviate from relaxed skin tension lines— nevertheless Langer's work remains the most important in any discussion regarding skin tension lines [16]. More recently, investigators studied porcine skin to assess the presence of 'Langer's Lines' and concluded that, as in humans, Langer's Lines do exist, and have specific patterns in pigskin [17] and are equally dynamic with movement—with the authors noting that in pigskin the "tension lines were oblique to the vertebra in the cephalic area, perpendicular to the vertebra in the middle torso, and parallel to the vertebra in the caudal area" [10]. One of the other factors that was considered prior to this testing was the relationship between Langer's Lines and hair follicles—experimental studies have shown that there is a good correlation between Langer's Lines and direction of hair streams [17] and this knowledge, hitherto help- ful in studying wounds, also helped in the design of this experiment—especially in the planning of skin markings and incisions for this study.

The mechanical theory of scalp whorl formation suggests that during the 10th to 17th week of fetal life, the brain expansion is so rapid that it creates a shearing force between the two layers of skin, at the dermo-epidermal junction, which in turn causes the hair follicles to curve [10]. While planning for this study, the author con- ducted expansion studies using saline expanders to understand the pressure required to create such shearing forces and the technique needed to replicate dermo-epidermal shear, and thereby the slanting of hair follicles. In a cross section of pigskin, as in Fig. 6.1 one can observe the epidermis and a layer of adipose tissue that serves as a fatty 'dermis' layer. Using saline expanders at the margins of pigskin cross-sections allowed us to observe dermo-epidermal shear. In this experiment, we found *rapid* expansion resulted in enough shearing force to separate the layers of skin. Slow expansion over hours, days or weeks did not result in creating enough 'shear' in pigskin to produce spirals. Pigskin has three separate fat layers, separated by two layers of fascia [18]. The uppermost layer of fat in pigskin corresponds to the der- mis in human skin—and authors have coined the term 'intradermal adipocytes' to describe these cells, as the term accurately reflects both their developmental origin and anatomical location [19]. Therefore, for the purposes of this experiment, the author decided to see if the causation of shearing forces between the uppermost two layers of pigskin (the epidermis and fatty dermis) would result in the formation of spirals along an advancing front.

6.2.2 The Experiment

Twenty freshly slaughtered pig bellies were obtained from an abattoir (supplied by FreshPork Northern, with the animals sourced from Timaru, New Zealand). Two parallel skin lines were marked along hair-follicle directions on pigskin, thereby

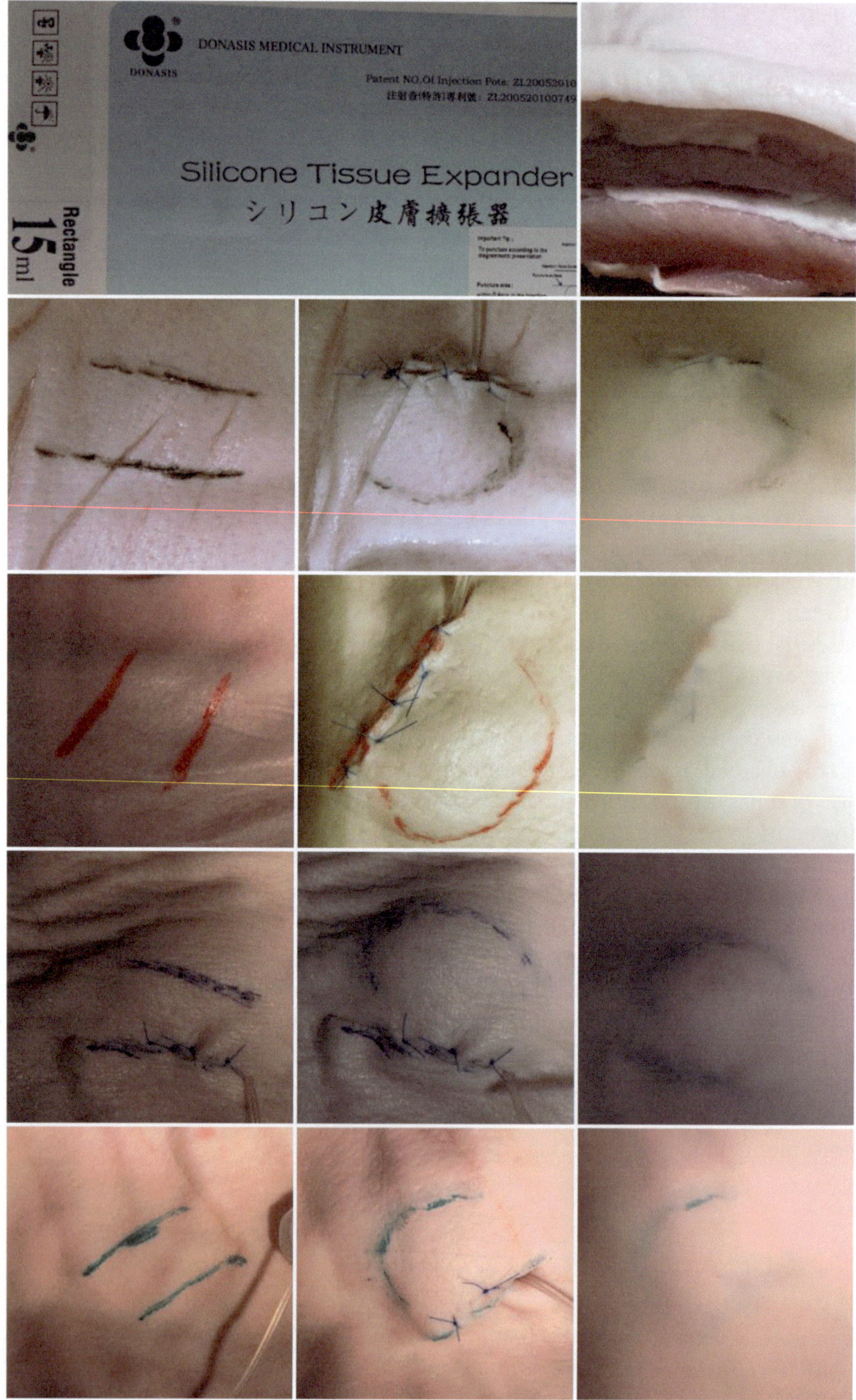

Fig. 6.1 Image shows saline expander, pigskin anatomy and curves formed by advancing front of rapid expansion

indicating two parallel skin tension lines, about 2 cm apart. These were marked along 'Langer's Lines' i.e. cleavage lines on the pig and not along wrinkle lines (photographs show that in some cases, wrinkle lines ran across the skin tension lines). Permanent indelible ink markers were used for each of these markings. A 15-mL silicone tissue expander was used in each case (Shanghai Wushan Industrial Co., Ltd., under license from Donasis Bio Labs, Japan). In this experiment, the author deliberately used a rectangular silicone expander to ensure that any spirals formed were not merely due to the shape of the implant used. A 2 cm incision was made in the skin, and was deepened to the muscle layer below the 'dermis' in the pig. A pocket was created, only wide enough to accommodate the collapsed silicone expander—just wide enough to fit the silicone expander that was firmly compressed and squashed into position. The incision was closed in layers. Care was taken to incorporate deeper layers within the deeper sutures to make sure that the 'advancing front' due to this rapid tissue expansion would be in one direction only (away from the suture-line) i.e. one of the two tension lines marked would be fixed to underlying tissues and not capable of expansion. The expanders were filled with saline rapidly (for purposes of this experiment, from previous testing, we defined this as expansion of the silicone expander with 10 mL of saline in under 2 s, followed by a further expansion to full capacity after 2 min). Tracing paper was placed over the pigskin and the curvature of the advancing line due to tissue expansion was marked out. The process was identical in each case, except we used a different pig belly in each case, and markings were traced using different coloured inks (Fig. 6.1).

The reason for the two-stage rapid expansion is because such staged protocols have been established in surgery for acute tissue expansion [20], with many authors supporting this method of rapid expansion to achieve additional skin cover during reconstructive surgery [21]. Further, during the testing phase, this study found this technique consistently caused enough dermo-epidermal shear to cause displacement of the fatty dermis and the creation of whorl patterns. During such acute expansion of tissue, biological and mechanical 'creep' occurs, and authors have postulated that it is the displacement of water from the collagen network and micro-fragmentation of elastic fibres that makes skin more viscous [22]. To mitigate any variability of technique and ensure accuracy, the same person (in this case the author) was the only person performing all the testing. The whole experiment was photographed and the images are published in his chapter.

6.3   Discussion

In our experiment, skin tracings of the advancing front (i.e. the non-sutured skin tension line that becomes deformed into curves under the force of rapid expansion) were marked out as detailed above (Fig. 6.1). To the naked eye, we could see that we had achieved some degree of displacement of the original straight-line markings into curves (Fig. 6.2). Interestingly, when we had traced out all the patterns and then superimposed all our tracings, one on top of each other to create a composite image,

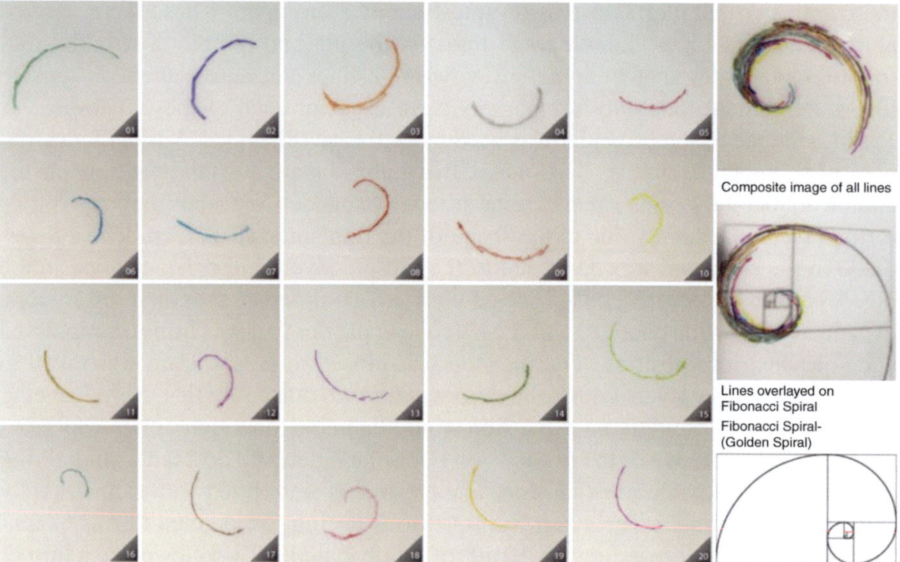

Fig. 6.2 Rapid expansion and skin line tracings—composite image created by overlaying tracings

we noted a distinctive logarithmic spiral pattern. The results are presented here—the composite image created by overlaying all our tracings show a clear logarithmic spiral pattern, in our case very close to a golden spiral pattern seen in nature. Figure 6.2 shows each individual tracing, followed by a composite image, finally overlaid by a golden spiral. Each tracing, when analyzed retrospectively did indeed conform to a portion of a golden spiral.

This experiment demonstrates clearly that under certain conditions, rapid tissue expansion causes dermo-epidermal shear, which can result in the formation of spirals—in our case, nature's own design: the golden spiral, perhaps nature's own design for *rapid* organic expansion.

As discussed earlier, spiral formations abound in nature and in tissues; they may represent a feature of rapid expansion along an advancing front. After all, the opening of flowers is often rapid—for example, Hedera helix, the English Ivy, opens in about 5 min [23], and many flowers demonstrate spiral patterns around their inflorescence axis. The opening of flowers is already known to be due to cellular expansion—while floral openings can be classified as nocturnal, diurnal, single or repetitive, previously published papers have demonstrated that the opening of flowers is generally due to cell expansion [23]. As to the genetics of such rapid expansion, researchers have studied rapid intraoperative tissue expansion in mouse skin and found that in response to stretch caused by a balloon, similar to our experiment, the following genes are induced—L1 (truncated long interspersed nucleotide element (1), myotubularin and insulin [24]. In another study on adult skin, researchers found a significant difference in 77 genes after expansion—with a significant finding being the expression of regeneration related genes, such as HOXA5, HOXB2 and AP1 after tissue expansion—with implications for further research into skin regeneration [25]. Indeed, studies in mono-zygotic twins have shown individual variations of scalp whorls, and therefore both skin stretch and the subsequent gene expression can be considered responsible for the formation of spirals [26].

Hakim and colleagues have studied spiral wave meander in excitable media and suggest that the dynamics of spiral waves can be reduced to a nonlinear equation of motion for the wave tip that is asymptotically exact in a parameter range where the motion takes place around a large central core region [27]. Other authors have studied the termination of pinned spirals on a defect by means of local stimuli [28]. When looked at conceptually, these findings are not unlike our findings in this experiment.

Knowledge gained from this experimental study has helped the author design a new technique for closing scalp defects based on the golden spiral where the motion takes place around a central core (measurements show cutaneous flaps raised in this way can stretch more than when raised in other shapes, and therefore can help in reconstruction of larger areas of scalp soft tissue), and this will be the subject the next section of this chapter.

The mechanical theory of scalp expansion causing whorls, while hypothesized, has never been re-created, to our knowledge, in a controlled experiment on skin. This study by this author that has been published previously [29] therefore represents a substantial advance in the understanding of both the formation of scalp whorls, skin biomechanics and specifically, the golden spiral pattern—which is widely found in galaxies and plants—and is probably nature's own design for rapid expansion of organic matter, along an advancing front. Given this this is an interesting and exciting new discovery, and may lead to further research in other fields of scientific endeavor, I have previously presented this to the wider scientific community beyond the surgical community [29].

6.4   The Golden Spiral Flap: A New Flap Design That Allows for Closure of Larger Scalp Wounds Better than Other Rotational Flap Designs

For the practice of surgery on skin, an understanding of skin lines is of paramount importance. Beginning with Langer's description [15] of 'cleavage lines' in 1861, many authors have studied and mapped out cutaneous 'skin tension' and wrinkle lines and adopted them for surgery. While understanding the tensile strength of a wound is important for wound closure [30], there has been poor scientific correlation between cutaneous wrinkle lines and wound tension. A team led by this author has used computational analyses to understand biodynamic excisional skin tension (BEST) lines i.e. the best lines of wound closure, after tissue has been removed by excision of skin lesions [31]. The study began on skin of the scalp for two reasons—it is relatively untethered to underlying tissues, and scalp whorls that appear to confirm to nature's golden spiral pattern are unique to human beings—and were thought to occur due to the rapid expansion of the brain during intrauterine life. While golden spiral patterns are evident in nature, there were considered mysterious until the study on skin mentioned above has suggested that this may indeed be nature's pattern for rapid expansion [29]. Such studies have recently demonstrated that when expansion of tissues was not rapid, whorl patterns did not result and that the golden spiral pattern may be useful as an intra-operative pattern for stretch [29]. It has also been established that biomechanically, skin behaves more like an elastic solid—a shell draped on a continuum foundation [32]. This continuum mechanics approach has shown to be of great use in understanding skin stretch, skin tension and tissue expansion, especially on sites like the scalp [33]. Also, the golden spiral pattern has previously been shown to be a pattern for rapid expansion of organic tissues [29]—and recent biomechanical studies on the scalp and the resultant mechanical theories all point to a continuum framework for finite growth [34, 35]. Studies therefore suggest that especially on the scalp, expansion and tension are interrelated, and the relationship between this stretch and expansion works like this: when skin is deformed either due to scalp expansion or stretch (as in the case of pivotal flaps), the deformation gradient has an elastic and a growth part [36].

The hypothesis that resulted as a corollary of this finding was that if the golden spiral pattern is nature's own grand design for rapid expansion, then the golden spiral could also be a method of stretching skin more efficiently during surgery—and this reduced wound tension would result in easier wound closure, stimulate growth factors and better wound healing. This experimental testing of this hypothesis, described below on pigskin and human skin, ultimately led to a new surgical method for scalp closure that is a major improvement on previous rotation flap techniques.

The scalp is a common site for the occurrence of skin cancer due to UV exposure and rotation flaps have been workhorses to reconstruct scalp defects after skin cancer excisions [37]. One of the main reasons to reduce tension in scalp flaps is the importance of maintaining perfusion pressure [38]. Throckmorton studied rotation flaps and the amount of flap stretch required to close defects, assuming a 2-dimensional surface and uniform 'deformation' of the flap during rotation. His studies found that for any incision longer than twice the diameter of the defect, the linear distance that the flap must be rotated ends up between 1.0 and 1.5 times the diameter of the defect; trigonometric analyses suggested that a ratio of 1.6:1 represented the ideal proportions of flap length to defect diameter [39]. When two rotation flaps were used from opposing directions on the scalp, optimal design is achieved by selecting a starting-point of the flap (on the defect) and creating a curvilinear flap with points 45° from each other at 2, 3, and 5 radii (Fig. 6.3). However, while 45° is the optimal angle for these flaps, undermining alone confers no advantage to decrease closing tension without accompanying flap incision, and flap-lengthening farther than 4 radii did not confer any advantage [40]. Closing the scalp without tension is important as tight closures in the scalp can lead to necrosis and skin loss which may in turn lead to more complicated bare-bone defects. Tight

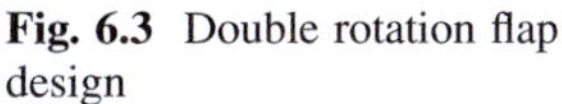

Fig. 6.3 Double rotation flap design

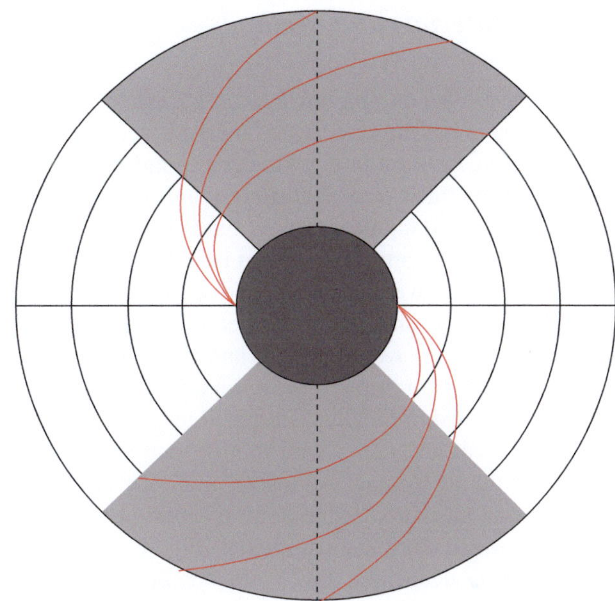

closures attempted by (otherwise useful) purse-string sutures on the scalp have led to scalp necrosis [41].

Semicircular geometric incisions have been often utilized as a method of closing scalp skin defects [42]. Single, double and triple pedicled rotational flaps have been described previously to close scalp skin defects, by pivoting skin about a base and sliding the semicircular skin flaps into place [37]. In general, these are hemi-circular pivotal flaps, and closure of a defect is performed by gently moving skin about a pivot, along the perimeter a circle. A series of experiments on rotational scalp tension concluded that tension was concentrated at 90° and 135°—in other words, extending the semicircle of the flap beyond 135° did not allow for easier closure [43].

While whorl and golden spiral patterns abound in nature in plants and space, on human scalp skin these whorls are significant for two reasons—every human has a scalp whorl, and these patterns are unique and different, even in twins [9]. The mechanical theory of scalp whorl formation suggests that during the 10th to 12th week of fetal life, the brain expansion is so rapid that it creates a shearing force between the two layers of skin, at the dermo-epidermal junction, which in turn causes the hair follicles to curve—resulting in the golden spiral pattern formation [10]. This remained a theory only, until recently, when a study by the author on pigskin replicated whorls by placing tissue under rapid stretch using saline tissue expanders, and re-creating rapid dermo-epidermal shear of skin [29].

To test the hypothesis that a golden spiral pattern therefore would be more efficient at expansion when compared to standard semicircular patterns, the author conducted a series of pigskin experiments. As the pigskin experiments demonstrated a significant reduction in tension using a golden spiral flap (as opposed to a traditional rotational flap), this was then validated by a clinical study on large scalp defects.

6.4.1 Materials and Methods

Pigskin was used as this has been established as the most comparable to human skin—pigskin has three separate fat layers, separated by two layers of fascia and the uppermost layer of fat in pigskin corresponds to the dermis in human skin [18].

Pigskin obtained from 20 different animals was tested as part of this study. The pigskin, freshly slaughtered, was obtained from an abattoir (supplied by FreshPork Northern, with the animals sourced from Timaru, New Zealand), and ten pig bellies and ten pig heads were used, so the results could be compared on different anatomical regions. One and two centimetre circular full-thickness defects (cutouts of fullthickness skin) were created, and flaps were created to close these defects—either using the traditional semicircular rotation flap design, or the golden spiral design. The pigskin blocks were glued to underlying boards using contact adhesive glue to prevent any underlying motion that could affect measurement (3 M 30NF Green Fastbond Contact Adhesive, manufactured by 3 M, St. Paul, MN, USA). Tension was measured at the point of maximum tension of the pivotal flaps, using a computerized digital tensiometer (Fig. 6.4) that has been used to study skin biodynamics, determine the biomechanical differences between 'tension' and 'relaxation' skin lines—and described in detail earlier [31]. This tensiometer, is ideal to study biomechanics of skin as it consists of a linear actuator, a force sensor, signal conditioning hardware and embedded software. To take a tension measurement the software starts by taking a calibration reading, this reading is known as the zero-tension point. The algorithm to calculate the tension ultimately is the differ-

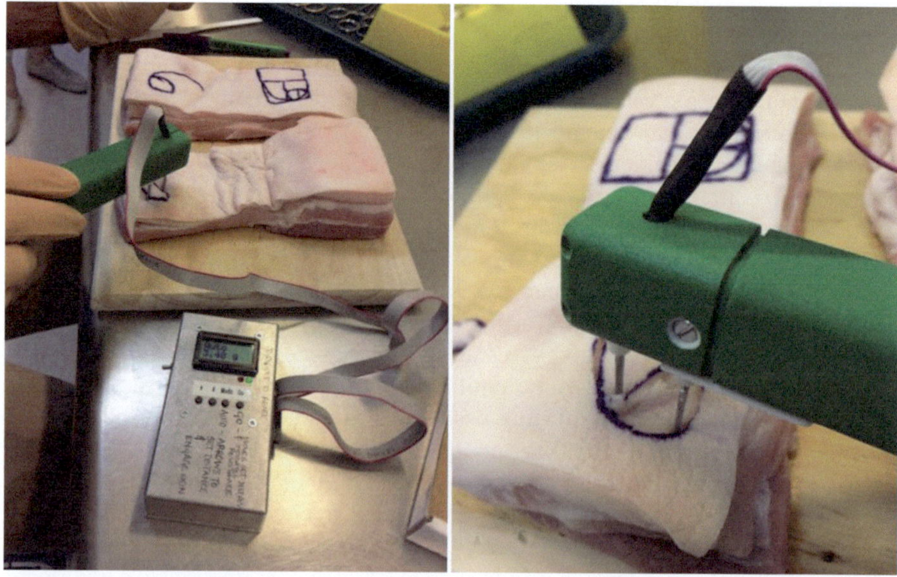

Fig. 6.4 Flap design tension comparisons using tensiometer on pigskin

ence between two force measurements as described above; these force measurements are derived from a digital ADC reading (0–1023) which is converted to grams using the formula (g = ADC value * 0.25), and these were converted to Newtons (N) for ease of publication of results. This device is bi-directional i.e. the user can measure inward and outward forces on scalp skin, and wound closing tension. This allows us to measure any inherent skin tension (pre-tension) and understand both skin tension and relaxation lines and details of this have been previously published [44].

The next stage of testing this hypothesis was formal study in patients, after obtaining all the necessary ethics approvals—New Zealand: Health and Disability Ethics Committee (HDEC Reference number 15/CEN/113); Australia: University of Queensland Institutional Human Ethics (Approval No. 2015001550). This study was carried out in accordance with the recommendations of ethics committees listed above, with written informed consent from all subjects. All subjects gave written informed consent in accordance with the Declaration of Helsinki. The results of the pigskin and clinical experiments are detailed below.

6.4.2   Results

The measurements, in the table below (Table 6.1) show the forces needed to close the wound using the two different flap techniques on pigskin.

The study showed that using the golden spiral flap allows us to close the wound under less tension, when compared to standard rotational flaps. The mean reduction in tension, in our study, was significant—at around 25%. A detailed statistical analysis was then undertaken by the mathematical sciences and statistics department that revealed the following: For both belly sites with a defect size ≥ 2 cm, and for head sites with defect size of 1 or 2 cm, the golden spiral method resulted in significantly less tension than the rotation flap method (one-sided pooled variance Student t test; $p = 0.0027$ (belly 2 cm), $p = 0.0043$ (head, 1 cm), $p = 0.00046$ (head, 2 cm)).

There were some interesting findings—when the wound was very small i.e. under 7 mm and the closing tension was low, there was not much difference between both the pivotal flap designs (Figs. 6.5 and 6.6)—and surgically-speaking, such wounds would be closed primarily without a flap anyway. Naturally, closing wounds on pig-heads needed greater force than the force needed to close softer pig-belly skin. However, as the defects became larger, the golden spiral flap proved much easier to close than a standard rotation flap, proving its superiority as a design capable of rapid stretch. During these pigskin experiments, it was noted that when conventional rotational flap designs were utilized, even the use of a back-cut reduced tension by less than 5%—and the golden spiral design facilitated much easier closure. This is because the golden spiral flap is in essence a logarithmic spiral flap with a growth factor of ϕ or the golden ratio [44]—what this means is that for every quarter turn the flap is rotated, it becomes progressively wider and therefore ends up closing wounds under less tension than a standard hemi-circular flap.

Table 6.1 Golden spiral and conventional rotational flap tension testing—force required to close the wound is recorded in Newtons (N)

No.	Site	Defect size (cm)	Rotation flap tension (N)	Golden spiral tension (N)	Variation %	Mean % reduction in tension
1	Belly	0.6	0.8	0.8	0	
2		0.7	1.0	1.0	0	
3		0.6	0.4	0.4	0	
4		0.7	0.8	0.8	0	
5		1	1.2	1.2	0	
6		2	1.6	1.2	−25	
7		2	2.0	1.3	−35	
8		2	2.1	1.2	−42.8	
9		2	1.5	1.2	−20	
10		2	2.7	2.0	−25.9	
11	Head	1	1.4	1.0	−28.5	
12		1	2.0	1.5	−25	
13		1	2.1	1.1	−47.6	
14		1	2.0	1.4	−30	
15		1	2.2	1.0	−54.5	
16		2	3.0	2.0	−33.3	
17		2	3.1	2.0	−35	
18		2	2.9	1.5	−48	
19		2	2.8	1.9	−32.1	
20		2	3.1	2.4	−22.5	
						25.2

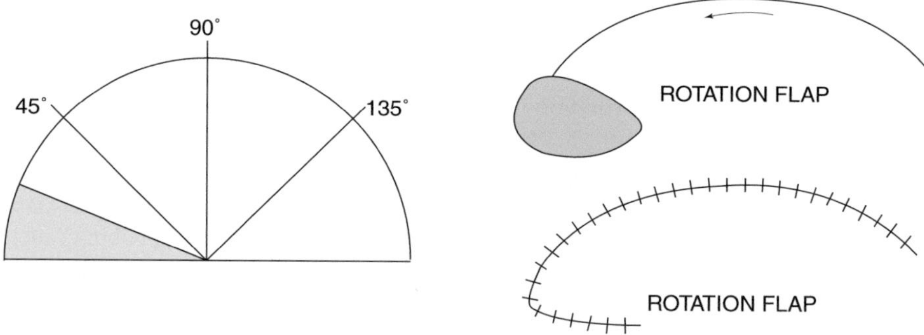

Fig. 6.5 Standard rotational flap design

The results presented, in this initial series of 11 patients, confirm our earlier impressions after pigskin testing: a flap based on the golden spiral pattern, nature's own design for expansion, achieves far superior results to a conventional semicircular rotational flap. Table 6.2 provides further details regarding the size and pathology of lesions that were excised. Most patients in this study needed excisions for skin cancer. The golden spiral flaps were planned, and tension measured (Fig. 6.7) as indicated in the clinical photographs—which show that even for 3 and 4 cm

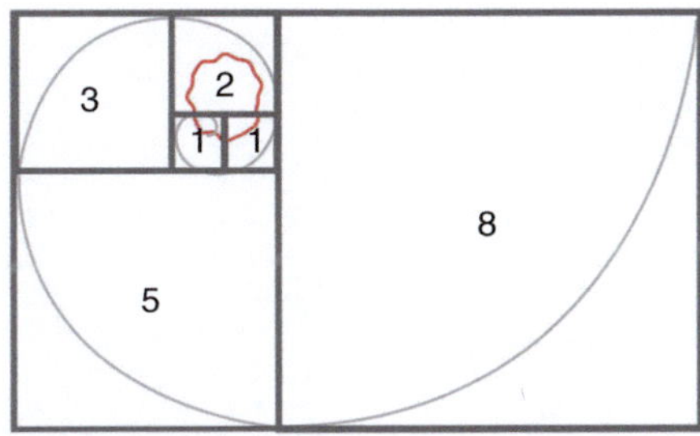
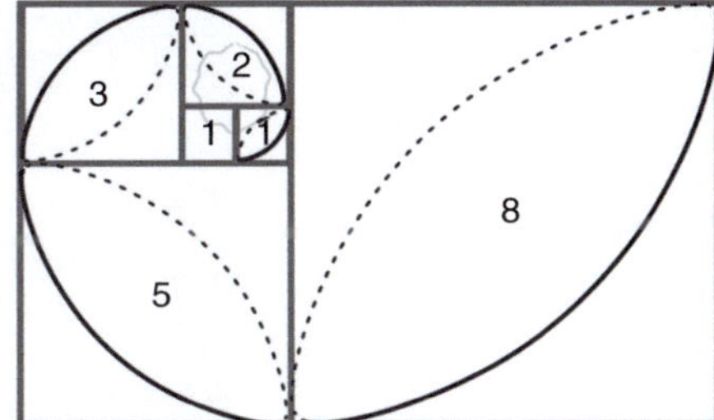

Fig. 6.6 Golden spiral flap design

Table 6.2 Pathology and size of lesions removed on the scalp

No.	Age	Sex	Diagnosis on histology	Diameter of defect (cm)	Site
1	88	M	Ulcer/post radiation necrosis	3	Scalp
2	50	F	BCC	3	Scalp
3	62	F	Trichilemmal cyst (proliferating)	4	Scalp
4	50	F	Basal cell cancer	3	Scalp
5	70	M	Squamous cell cancer	2	Scalp
6	68	M	Squamous cell cancer	4	Scalp
7	70	M	Basal cell cancer	2.5	Scalp
8	70	M	Basal cell cancer	2	Scalp
9	68	M	Basal cell cancer	3	Scalp
10	88	M	Squamous cell cancer	2.5	Scalp
11	65	M	Hypertrophic actinic keratosis	2	Scalp

defects, closure was achieved relatively easily (Figs. 6.8 and 6.9). Even though the defects ranged from 2 to 4 cm, closure was achieved without tension or the need for skin grafting. There were no wound complications (infection or dehiscence) in this series. The author notes, on viewing the final result after wound closure, that the golden spiral flap may appear to have a narrower pedicle than one might expect for this design, but this did not result in any flap necrosis or wound complications. We can conclude therefore that while the design is similar to a rotational flap, the golden spiral flap is indeed a different kind of a random-pattern pivotal flap that is especially usefully on the scalp—where random-pattern flaps, nourished by large blood vessels located in the subcutaneous layer just superficial to the galea aponeurosis, are especially useful.

6.5 Discussion

The golden spiral flap presented here is a valuable new addition to a surgeon's armamentarium when faced with large scalp defects, especially after skin cancer. Given the ease of using the sequential-Fibonacci-squares method to mark out the flap, it is adaptable to defects of various sizes easily. In general, the defect will lie

Fig. 6.7 Scalp tension mea-surement during surgery

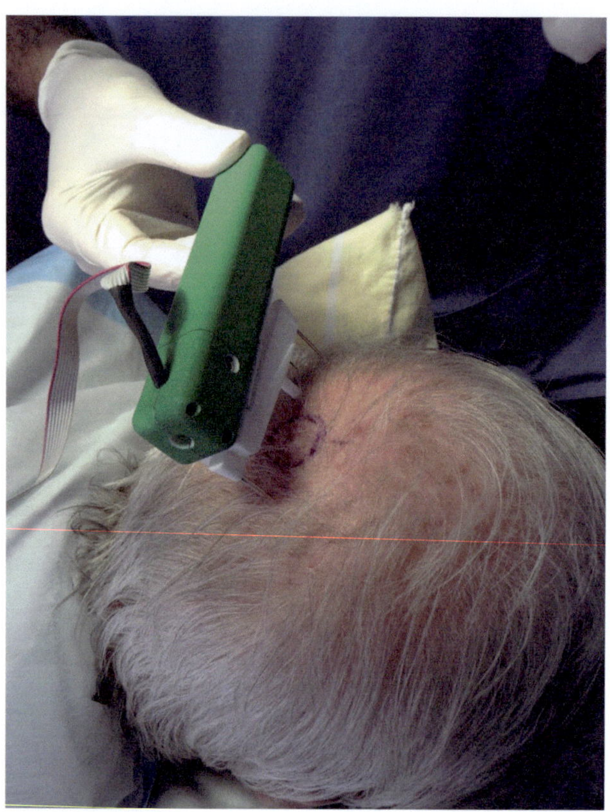

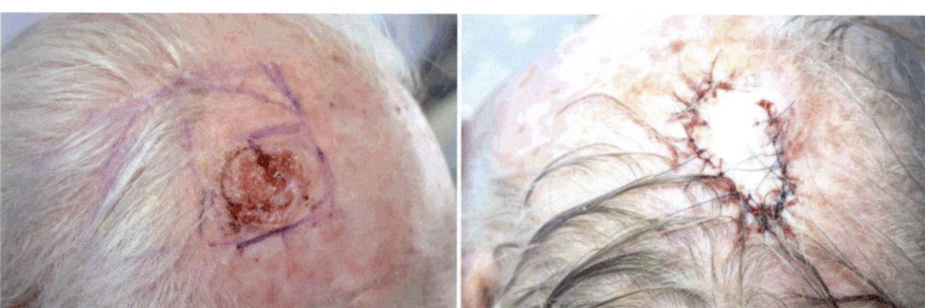

Fig. 6.8 Golden spiral flaps (1)

within the first three squares, but given the nature of the design it is extremely adaptable. The dissection and undermining is done similar to other cutaneous flaps on the scalp, with dissection down to the loose areolar tissue. We have found that utilizing the golden spiral pattern on skin to be safe and reliable, with the added benefit of progressively lowered tension while closing larger defects. The main application of this random-pattern pivotal golden spiral flap will be to facilitate

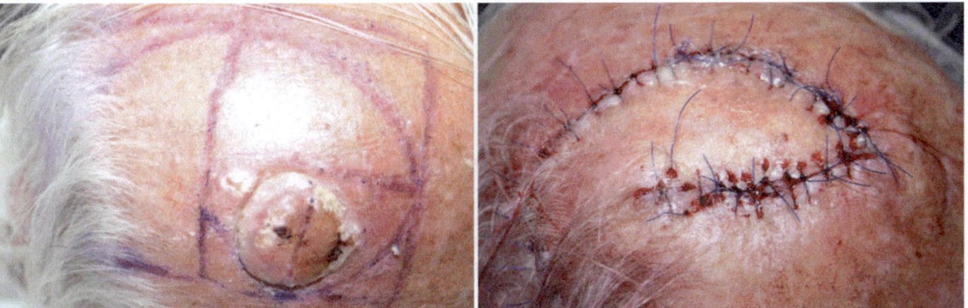

Fig. 6.9 Golden spiral flaps (2)

closure of large scalp wounds where primary closure is not feasible. However, even if the biomechanics have only been studied on the scalp, it is likely to be useful on other sites on the head and neck where one does not need a perforator-based flap. While the primary interest of this paper will be to a medical, dental or veterinary audience, the author notes with interest that spiral patterns are increasingly studied in other media—Hakim and colleagues have studied spiral wave meander in excitable media and suggest that the dynamics of spiral waves can be reduced to a nonlinear equation of motion for the wave tip that is asymptotically exact in a parameter range—where the motion takes place around a large central core region [27]. Other authors have studied the termination of pinned spirals on a defect by means of local stimuli [45]. This study and the development of the Golden Spiral Flap design has been published previously by this author [46]. When looked at conceptually, studies on spiral patterns from other industries also demonstrate the utility of the golden spiral pattern as a pattern for rapid expansion—and this experiment may be of interest to both the wider scientific community, and of course, a surgical audience [46].

References

1. Naylor M. Golden, $\sqrt{2}$, and ϕ flowers: a spiral story. Math Mag. 2002;75(3):163–72.
2. Catrakis HJ. The logarithmic spiral: mathematical aspects and modeling in turbulence. J Math Res. 2011;3(3):3–11.
3. Ingrouille M. Steps up the botanic spirals. Nat Book Rev. 1994;369(7052):718.
4. Spirals in nature. J Franklin Inst. 1993;15(3):352.
5. Natural spirals. Nature. 2005;436(7052):757.
6. Ma J, et al. Simulating the formation of spiral wave in the neuronal system. Nonlinear Dyn. 2013;73(1–2):73–83.
7. Li C, Ji A, Cao Z. Stressed Fibonacci spiral patterns of definite chirality. Appl Phys Lett. 2007;90(16):164102.
8. Leung KT, Józsa L, Ravasz M, Néda Z. Pattern formation: spiral cracks without twisting. Nature. 2001;410(6825):166.
9. Wunderlich RC, Heerema NA. Hair crown patterns of human newborns. Studies on parietal hair whorl locations and their directions. Clin Pediatr. 1975;14(11):1045–9.

10. Samlaska CP, James WD, Sperling LC. Scalp whorls. J Am Acad Dermatol. 1989;21(3 Pt 1):553–6.
11. Randle H, Webb TG, Gill LJ. The relationship between facial hair whorls and temperament in Lundy ponies. Annu Rep Lundy Field Soc. 2003;52:67–83.
12. Herron AJ. Pigs as dermatologic models of human skin disease. In: Proceeding of the ACVP/ASVCP concurrent annual meetings 5–9 Dec 2009, Monterey, CA.
13. Schmook FP, Meingassner JG, Billich A. Comparison of human skin or epidermis models with human and animal skin in in-vitro percutaneous absorption. Int J Pharm. 2001;215(1–2):51–6.
14. Gibson T. Editorial Karl Langer (1819–1887) and his lines. Br J Plast Surg. 1978;3(1):1–2.
15. Langer K. On the anatomy and physiology of the skin I. The cleavability of the cutis. Br J Plast Surg. 1978;31(1):3–8.
16. Borges AF. Relaxed skin tension lines (RSTL) versus other skin lines. Plast Reconstr Surg. 1984;73(1):144–50.
17. Kwak M, Son D, Kim J, Han K. Static Langer's line and wound contraction rates according to anatomical regions in a porcine model. Wound Repair Regen. 2014;22(5):678–82.
18. Anderson DB, Kauffman RG, Kastenschmidt LL. Lipogenic enzyme activities and cellularity of porcine adipose tissue from various anatomical locations. J Lipid Res. 1972;13(5):593–9.
19. Driskell RR, Jahoda CA, Chuong CM, Watt FM, Horsley V. Defining dermal adipose tissue. Exp Dermatol. 2014;23(9):629–31.
20. Chandawarkar R, et al. Intraoperative acute tissue expansion revisited: a valuable tool for challenging skin defects. Dermatol Surg. 2003;29(8):834–8.
21. Sasaki GH. Intraoperative sustained limited expansion (ISLE) as an immediate reconstructive technique. Clin Plast Surg. 1987;14(3):563–73.
22. Wilhelmi BJ, Blackwell SJ, Mancoll JS, Phillips LG. Creep vs. stretch: a review of the viscoelastic properties of skin. Ann Plast Surg. 1998;41(2):215–9.
23. Van Doorn WG, et al. Flower opening and closure: a review. J Exp Bot. 2003;54(389):1801–12.
24. Zhu Y, Barker J, et al. Identification of genes induced by rapid intraoperative tissue expansion in mouse skin. Arch Dermatol Res. 2002;293(11):560–8.
25. Yang M, et al. A preliminary study of differentially expressed genes in expanded skin and normal skin: implications for adult skin regeneration. Arch Dermatol Res. 2011;303(2):125–33.
26. Paine ML, et al. Hair whorls and monozygosity. J Invest Dermatol. 2004;122(4):1057.
27. Hakim V, Karma A. Spiral wave meander in excitable media: the large core limit. Phys Rev Lett. 1997;79(4):665.
28. Jiang-Xing C, Ming-Ming G, Jun M. Termination of pinned spirals by local stimuli. Europhys Lett. 2016;113(3)
29. Paul SP. Golden spirals and scalp whorls: nature's own design for rapid expansion. PLoS One. 2016;11(9):e0162026.
30. Milch RA. Tensile strength of surgical wounds. J Surg Res. 1965;5:77–385.
31. Paul SP, Matulich J, Charlton NA. New skin tensiometer device: computational analyses to understand biodynamic excisional skin tension lines. Sci Rep. 2016;6:30117.
32. Danielson DA. Wrinkling of the human skin. J Biomech. 1977;10(3):201–4.
33. Zollner AM, Buganza Tepole A, Gosain AK, Kuhl E. Growing skin: tissue expansion in pediatric forehead reconstruction. Biomech Model Mechanobiol. 2012;11(6):855–67.
34. Buganza Tepole A, Gosain AK, Kuhl E. Stretching skin: the physiological limit and beyond. Int J Non Linear Mech. 2011;47(8):938–49.
35. Rodriguez EK, Hoger A, McCulloch AD. Stress-dependent finite growth in soft elastic tissues. J Biomech. 1994;27:455–67.
36. Garikipati K. The kinematics of biological growth. Appl Mech Rev. 2009;62(3):030801.
37. Paul SP, Norman RA. Rotation flaps of the scalp: study of the design, planning and biomechanics of single, double and triple pedicle flaps. Clinical cases in skin cancer surgery and treatment. Cham: Springer; 2016. p. 31–44.
38. Cutting C. Critical closing and perfusion pressures in flap survival. Ann Plast Surg. 1982;9:524.

39. Throckmorton GS, Williams FC, Potter JK, Finn R. The geometry of skin flap rotation. J Oral Maxillofac Surg. 2010;68:2545–8.
40. Buckingham ED, Quinn FB, Calhoun KH. Optimal design of O-to-Z flaps for closure of facial skin defects. Arch Facial Plast Surg. 2003;5(1):92–5.
41. Cohen PR, Martinelli PT, Schulze KE, et al. The purse-string suture revisited: a useful technique for the closure of cutaneous surgical wounds. Int J Dermatol. 2007;46:341–7.
42. Costa DJ, Walen S, Varvares M, Walker RJ. Scalp rotation flap for reconstruction of complex soft tissue defects. J Neurol Surg B Skull Base. 2016;77(1):32–7.
43. Larrabee WF, Sutton D. The biomechanics of advancement and rotation flaps. Laryngoscope. 1981;91(5):726–44.
44. Mukhopadhyay U. Logarithmic spiral—a splendid curve. Resonance. 2004;9(11):39–45.
45. Chen J-X, Guo M-M, Ma J. Termination of pinned spirals by local stimuli. EPL. 2016; 113(3):38004.
46. Paul SP. The golden spiral flap: a new flap design that allows for closure of larger wounds under reduced tension – how studying nature's own design led to the development of a new surgical technique. Front Surg. 2016;3:63. https://doi.org/10.3389/fsurg.2016.00063

Chapter 7
Breaking up BEST Lines Using Zigs and Zags: Lengthening *v.* Reduction of Tension

7.1 Introduction

The sternal region and the intra-mammary region has been the bane of many a cutaneous surgeon, with a higher propensity for poor scarring and wound complications. West and others coined the term "keloid triangle" to indicate the suprasternal region where scars become especially conspicuous and prone to hypertrophic and keloid scarring [1]. To these regions, we should add the cervicomandibular region and the cervicothoracic regions (Fig. 7.1). While the chest wall is exposed to multiple shearing forces due to limb movements, the weight of breast tissue also contributes to scar stretch and increased wound tension. The resultant mechanics of scar mechanotransduction, a term that has come to denote the conversion of mechanical stimuli into biochemical responses at different body sites remain unclear, and ultimately the resultant scar is largely determined by the biomechanical properties of skin itself [2, 3]. In humans and mammals, wounds heal by fibrotic scar formation, which provides early restoration of tissue integrity, as opposed to the functional regeneration that occurs in lower animals [4]. The continuum mechanics approach has shown to be of great use in understanding skin stretch, skin tension, and tissue expansion, especially on sites close to the bone such as the sternum and areas like the scalp [5]. When skin is stretched during the closure phase of excisional surgery, its expansion and tension are interrelated, and the relationship between this stretch and expansion works like this: the deformation gradient has an elastic and a growth part and therefore it is important to understand the biomechanics of skin tension at different sites and the signals it generates [6]. This signal of mechanotransduction involves proteins and molecules of the ECM, the cytoplasmic and nuclear membranes and the cytoskeleton, eventually affecting the nuclear chromatin at a genetic level [7]. The system that brings together all the levels of mechanotransduction and their influence on genetic cell programming has been termed "tensegrity," a portmanteau of tension and integrity [8].

© Springer International Publishing AG, part of Springer Nature 2018

S. P. Paul, *Biodynamic Excisional Skin Tension Lines for Cutaneous Surgery*,

https://doi.org/10.1007/978-3-319-71495-0_7

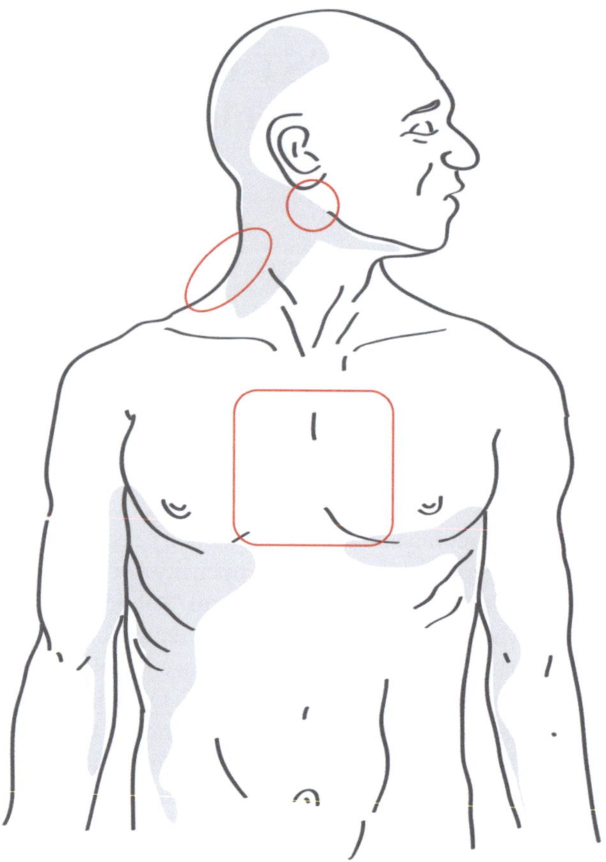

Fig. 7.1 Well known keloid zones on the body

Many groups have studied models of scarring using external application of mechanical stress on healing incisions—as mechanical force is the major factor in fibro proliferative processes that cause tissue fibrosis and hypertrophic scarring [9]. Porcine skin anatomy is like human skin, and therefore pig models have been used by many authors to study human cutaneous mechanobiology, including in this study [2]. Gurtner and others have shown that scar formation in the red Duroc pig is very like that in humans, and the degree of post-injury fibrosis *directly* correlates with the amount of tension imparted on the wound during healing, and this fact influenced our choice of medium for this study [10]. While mechanotransduction involves stretch activated calcium-dependent ion channels [11], the tension in the wound generates cell traction forces in the cellular cytoskeleton that are then transmitted to the surrounding ECM or neighbouring cells [12].

Initial observations on keloid scars were made in burn wounds, with researchers noting that a wound that healed under 10 days had only 4% risk of developing hypertrophic scarring, whereas when a burn took 3 weeks to heal, the risk rises to 70% [13]. We know that the characteristic butterfly or dumbbell shape associated with keloids is determined by the direction of mechanical forces, and therefore an understanding of these forces, and reduction of wound tension is of great importance to reduce scar formation [14]. Authors of studies of mechanical forces on skin have concluded that reducing skin tension around wounds or scars is the most important step in reducing thick, unsightly scars [15].

The other approach to reducing the visibility of scars has been using a visual approach, rather than a mechanical one—proponents of geometric broken line repairs have written that such closures make "the scar less noticeable because the eye has more difficulty tracking this irregular, multiply segmented line [16]." But a review of the neuroscience of vision and optical illusions does not back up this claim. In fact, preliminary studies into sharp broken lines, that occur after a Z-plasty or zigzag surgical procedure, suggest that they may be less pleasing to the eye. This was first noted in an important study by Stratton who used participants viewing different types of lines, only to conclude that eye movements that are required to follow sharp, broken lines must be more abrupt and, therefore, less pleasant than those required to follow curved lines [17]. On the other hand, some authors have proposed that zigzag lines indeed appear mobile and less visible in peripheral visual fields, and that a short line segment squirms along a zigzag line, even if this is only when viewed in one's peripheral vision [18]. In fact, certain authors have hypothesized an evolutionary origin to the visualization of sharp broken lines as a perception of danger or unpleasantness (shark teeth, for example) [19]. However, others have noted that when proposing an evolutionary origin, it is not enough to suggest a plausible explanation but a testable hypothesis is required [20]. That may be the best approach to take when planning excisional surgery in "keloid-zones" of the body. It has already been established that the most important factor to reduce scarring in scar-prone areas is the reduction of the maximal wound tension, and in this chapter the author undertakes a review of different methods of breaking up scars by utilizing zigs and zags—and the implications for surgical wound-closing tension. A pigskin study conducted into the use of the simple zigzag to reduce the tension (and thereby scarring) of surgical wounds is reported here, and a comparison undertaken with elliptical excision and Z-plasties (Fig. 7.2).

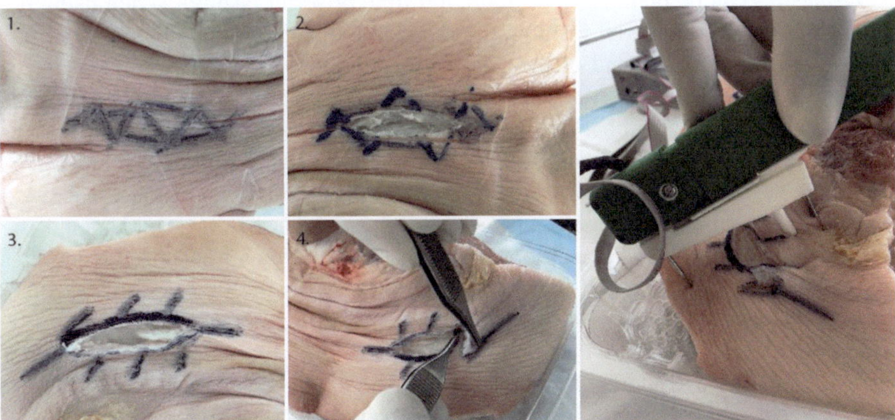

Fig. 7.2 Wound tension testing of zigzags and Z-plasties on pigskin

7.2 Z-Plasty

The history of the Z-plasty is rooted in oculoplastic surgery. The first recorded case was when William Horner, a surgeon at the Philadelphia Hospital, Blockley and Professor of Anatomy at the University of Pennsylvania, performed this procedure to repair an eyelid ectropion caused by burn scarring [21]. However, some reports attribute the first Z-plasty to Denonvilliers, who noted the usefulness of breaking up a scar-line into zigs and zags when he first described a Z-plasty–type procedure that he found useful, also for a blepharoplasty [22]. Denonvilliers had written about his plan thus: "I will free the lowered external angle of the eye by two incisions above and below the lid margins meeting at the angle. Then I will form above and a little external to the first triangle, a second triangle opposite to the first. This accomplished, I will raise the triangle involving the external corner of the eye and cause it to take the place of the second triangle that I will then bring down to take the place of the first" [23]. While this complicated description seems apt for a Z-plasty, there were no physical illustrations or images to record the procedure. Stewart McCurdy, an American surgeon, then utilized the same method for the oral commissure. McCurdy, who was Professor of Oral and General Surgery at the University of Pittsburgh, and Orthopaedic and Plastic Surgeon to Columbia and Presbyterian Hospitals is credited as being the first one to use the term "Z-plasty" when he published his article: "Z-plastic surgery: plastic operations to elongate cicatricial contractions of the neck, lips and eyelids and across joints [24]." Limberg, in 1966, famed for his rhombic flaps [25], also wrote extensively on the Z-plasty, although it would seem Limberg considered the term a misnomer—given that in the alphabetical "Z" all the limbs are equal, unlike in surgical versions [26]. Limberg favoured the term "transposed triangular flaps" [27] to describe this technique, and later in his book described a full range of such procedures from equal-angled flaps (where each flap moves equally), to flaps with unequal angles (where the larger angled flap moves less) [28]. However, McCurdy's term, "Z-plasty" endured the test of time.

Z–plasties can be planned in a single, multiple or serial fashion. When using the multiple Z-plasty in a serial fashion, the planned incisions run parallel to the limbs of the Z-plasty at either end of the scar. In this chapter I am describing the use of zigs and zags to reduce sternal scarring, and indeed scarring at other flexural areas at the jawline, neck or limbs. But using a Z-plasty in this situation can be problematic due to the lengthening it causes. Further, with the serial Z-plasty technique, as would be needed in a location such as the sternum, the flaps become three-sided rhombic flaps, and not two-sided triangles. Now we can begin to understand the wisdom of Limberg's insistence of calling the procedure as transposed triangular flaps. Also, it must be noted that the limbs in between the two peripheral limbs become approximately twice the length of the limbs before transposition. Essentially, when it comes to a Z-plasty the angles of the limbs are important—it is known that using 30° angles will increase the length by 25%, 45° angles are associated with a 50% increase and 60° angles increase the ideal length by 75% [29].

Let's consider a triangle with sides a, b and c (and opposing angles A, B and C). In any triangle, if sides a and b and the angle C are known, then side c can be found by using the following formula [30]:

$$c^2 = a^2 + b^2 - 2ab\left[\cos C\right]$$

And, if the three sides a, b and c are known, then we find angle A using the following formula:

$$\cos A = \left(b^2 + c^2 - a^2\right)/2bc$$

Using these formulas, we arrive at the conclusion that in a 60° Z-plasty, the common limb rotates by 90°. Figure 7.3 shows the degree of rotation of the common limb, and helps us design the correct Z-plasty depending on the location of the scar from a crease-line, and the degree of rotation needed to hide the scar. When it comes to Z-plasties where no lengthening is required, such as over the sternal region, the purpose of the Z is to equalize tension, with the preferred angle being 30° for each limb of the Z.

Furnas described the four features of a Z-plasty thus [31]:

1. To increase (or decrease) length
2. To break up a straight line
3. To shift topographic features from one site to another
4. To efface or to create a web or a cleft

However, one of the things to note in a Z-plasty is—the wider the angles of the triangular flaps, the greater is the tension on the line of closure. In areas like the sternum, if we consider using a Z-plasty to break up a scar, we are left with the problem of alteration in length, as well as tension on the line of closure to consider. The fundamental benefit of a Z-plasty is its ability to lengthen a limb, and therefore correct a contracture. While plenty of studies have elucidated the angles and degrees of rotation and lengthening, there have been none that have specifically studied the reduction of tension in using a Z-plasty and that will be the focus of this review. There is an important matter to consider regarding Z-plasty in areas of thin, actinic-damaged skin on the face or burn scar contractures, as opposed to scar-prone

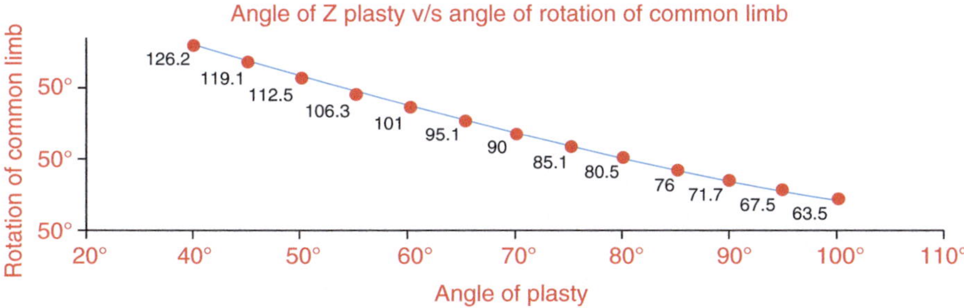

Fig. 7.3 Z-plasty: angles and degrees of rotation

areas on the chest. In the former, maximizing blood flow to the flaps is also a major objective; in the latter, the main consideration is reducing skin stress and tension. Some surgeons have suggested "rhomboid-to-W" technique, incorporating a W-plasty into other rhomboid defects or triangular flaps, and therefore this review will look at a W-plasty in the next section.

7.3   W-Plasty

When Borges elucidated the W-plasty technique, he basically considered the benefits as fourfold [32]:

1. Breaking up of the scar into smaller components
2. Redirecting anti-tension lines
3. Halving the depth i.e. the subcutaneous scar does not coincide with the zigzag cutaneous scar
4. Camouflaging scar by intermingling these small segments with other skin creases and wrinkles

The W-plasty has proved to be very useful in areas like vermillion [33] or mental creases, has also been used in tracheal reconstruction [34], to repair stoma stenosis [35] and to break up scars of rotation flaps on the cheek [36]. The W-plasty is primarily useful around labial regions, both oral [37] and perineal [38]. It has also been used primarily during repair of lacerations in these sites [37]. However, when used as a means of primary closure after excisional of a lesion in a keloid zone, it involves removal of additional tissue in an area already prone to tension and that is its disadvantage.

7.4   Geometric Broken-Line Closure (GBLC)

Any scar revision technique must be based on risk/reward assessment. Some authors have suggested that scars 2 cm in length or scars greater than 2 mm in width can be improved by geometric broken line closures [39]. One of the first people to describe Geometric Broken Line Closure (GBLC) was Wessberg in 1982 [40]. The technique of GBLC is as the name indicates—the scar is excised using geometric lines, drawn in such a fashion that triangles, rectangles, and squares are created in a random pattern (Fig. 7.2). The main rationale in this technique is that converts a long, easily visible scar into a scar broken up into multiple short segments, and it is said that the scar becomes less apparent because the human eye has more difficulty tracking an irregular, multiply segmented line as opposed to a thicker straight line [41]. Studies have been done on pre-sternal scars after cardiothoracic surgery to understand this predisposition to cause hypertrophic scarring, with studies confirming that scars on the sternum especially in women, tend to hypertrophy (even when there is no keloid tendency) after incisional wounds [42]. The main biomechanical issue on the sternal region is that the tension acts equally in all directions and this results in a higher risk of hypertrophic scarring [43]. In other areas on the body close to bone, skin exhibits not just anisotropy, but also orthotropy i.e. directional symmetry [44]. This degree of symmetry with respect to two normal planes is thought to be due to the preferential orientation of collagen fibres [7]. Breaking up a scar in smaller segments in differing directions therefore helps reduce the pull on the scar, thereby reducing the risk of hypertrophic scar formation.

But the GBLC is problematic outside the face region, from a technical point of view. For a start, it is usually employed to correct existing scars, not prevent them, and it is generally accepted among plastic surgeons "that the scar should be greater than 30° off the RSTL [45]." As we are discussing the use of zigs and zags in incisional surgery to reduce the risk of hypertrophic and keloid scarring, it seems out of place. However, the clincher seems to be this for an area like the sternum that is already prone to problematic scarring—as Shockley notes, "Because additional excision of normal tissue is required, the GBLC technique should only be considered in areas where there is sufficient skin redundancy and elasticity for closure without tension [46]." The dermal structures of the chest and sternum by themselves confer an additional risk of scarring. As noted in studies by other authors, the anterior chest is the most frequent keloid-bearing site on the body; however, the anterior chest is not the site with the most frequent stretching/contraction—suggesting that other than skin mobility, it is indeed high tension with cyclical stretching that matters the most [15]. Other than respiration, the tension caused by coughing may also cause wound problems. It has been noted that a normal cough reaches 100 mmHg, producing a force of 56 kg, whereas a forceful cough can generate a pressure of 300 mmHg, and produce a force of 168 kg [47]. Others have developed mathematical models of sternotomy wounds to calculate the force generated by coughing and other stressors on a chest wound [48]:

$$T = rlP = 0.17 \ m \times 0.25 \ m \times 5.6 \ kPa = 238 \ N \sim 24 \ kg$$

The chest is also a unique location from a biodynamic point of view because when people pull their chest in, the horizontal stretching/contraction rates are greater than the vertical; whereas, when people raise their hands, the vertical and oblique stretching rates are greater than the horizontal rates and this creates both constant and variable tension [49]. And, given we have been discussing that reduction of tension is the most important factor in reducing scarring, given the multidirectional stressors, these become important considerations.

7.5   The Simple Zigzag to Reduce Tension Over Keloid Zones

A review undertaken of the different zigs and zags in use to improve scarring demonstrated the benefits of breaking up a scar into smaller segments. However, when used during primary closure, the techniques have some clear differences—the Z-plasty is all about angles, degrees of rotation and lengthening (Figs. 7.3 and 7.4), while the W-plasty and the geometric broken line closure involve cutting out additional tissue on both sides of the wound (Fig. 7.5). The geometric broken line

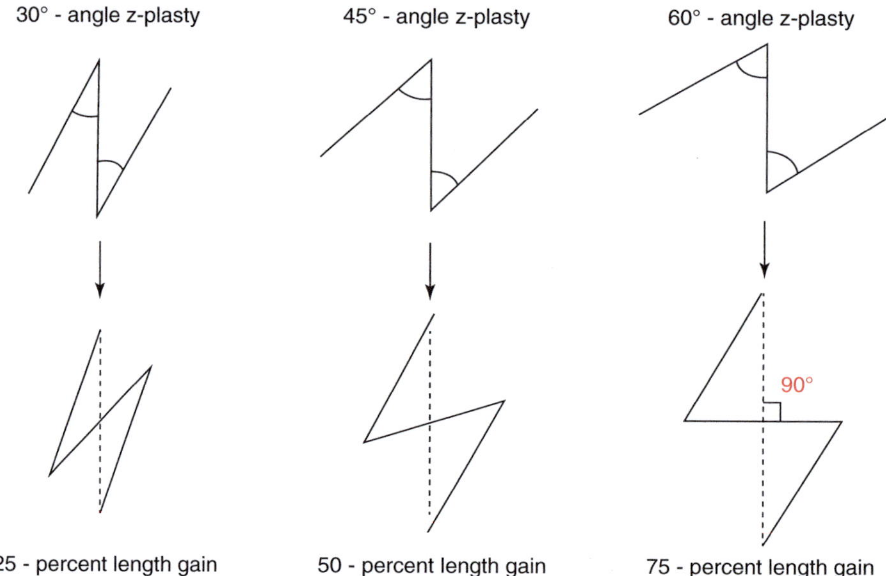

Fig. 7.4 Z-plasty: angles and lengthening that occurs

Fig. 7.5 Geometric Broken Line Closure (GBLC) and W-plasty

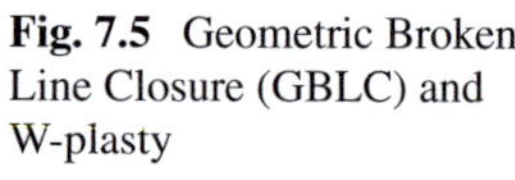

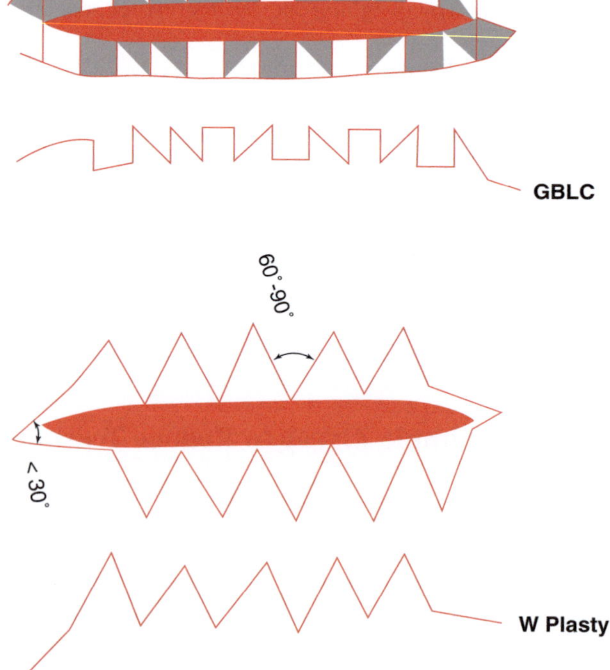

closure is difficult to perform during a primary elliptical excision and more suited to a scar revision of a thick cicatrix. The author therefore pondered if using a simple zigzag would be of benefit during primary elliptical excision in a keloid-prone zone? There were two questions that needed answering:

1. Would a zigzag excision cause a reduction in mechanical forces which we already know is the major factor in fibro-proliferative processes that cause tissue fibrosis and hypertrophic scarring?
2. How does a zigzag compare biomechanically with a Z-plasty i.e. are all zigzags created equal?

7.6   Materials and Methods

A series of 30 elliptical wounds created on pigskin were assigned into three groups of ten each. Each comparison was done on identical pigskin i.e. the same animal. Ten standard elliptical closures, ten Z-plasties of 30° and ten simple zigzag excisions were done (Figs. 7.2 and 7.6). The simple zigzag also had a 30° angle in our study. Tension measurements were taken using a previously described and studied tensiometer [50]. The first reading was at the midpoint because authors have previously noted that the closing tension perpendicular to any linear incision is a function of the incision's length and is maximal at the midpoint of the length [51]. To obtain a clear understanding, readings were taken at three points (marked 1, 2, 3 in Fig. 7.6). These points were—the midpoint of the ellipse where tension was expected to be maximal, one end of the excision and a third reading taken midway between the two points just mentioned.

The tension measurements were noted, as was any lengthening that occurred of the wound. The results were overseen by the mathematical sciences and statistics department who performed a detailed statistical analysis.

7.7   Results

Measurements of tension taken were as follows in Newtons (N) (Fig. 7.6):

m1 (simple ellipse) = (2.3, 2.0, 2.2, 1.8, 1.9, 2.3, 1.9, 2.3, 1.0, 2.0)
m2 (Z-plasty) = (2.0, 1.8, 2.0, 2.0, 1.8, 1.7, 1.9, 1.9, 1.7, 1.4)
m3 (simple zigzag) = (2.0, 1.8, 1.5, 0.9, 1.0, 1.6, 1.3, 1.6, 1.2, 1.0)
Mean tension measurements (N) were least in the simple zigzag:
mean(m1) 1.97
mean(m2) 1.82
mean(m3) 1.39

In the case of the simple elliptical closure of the simple zigzag excision, no lengthening of the wound was noted. In the Z-plasty lengthening was noted, in

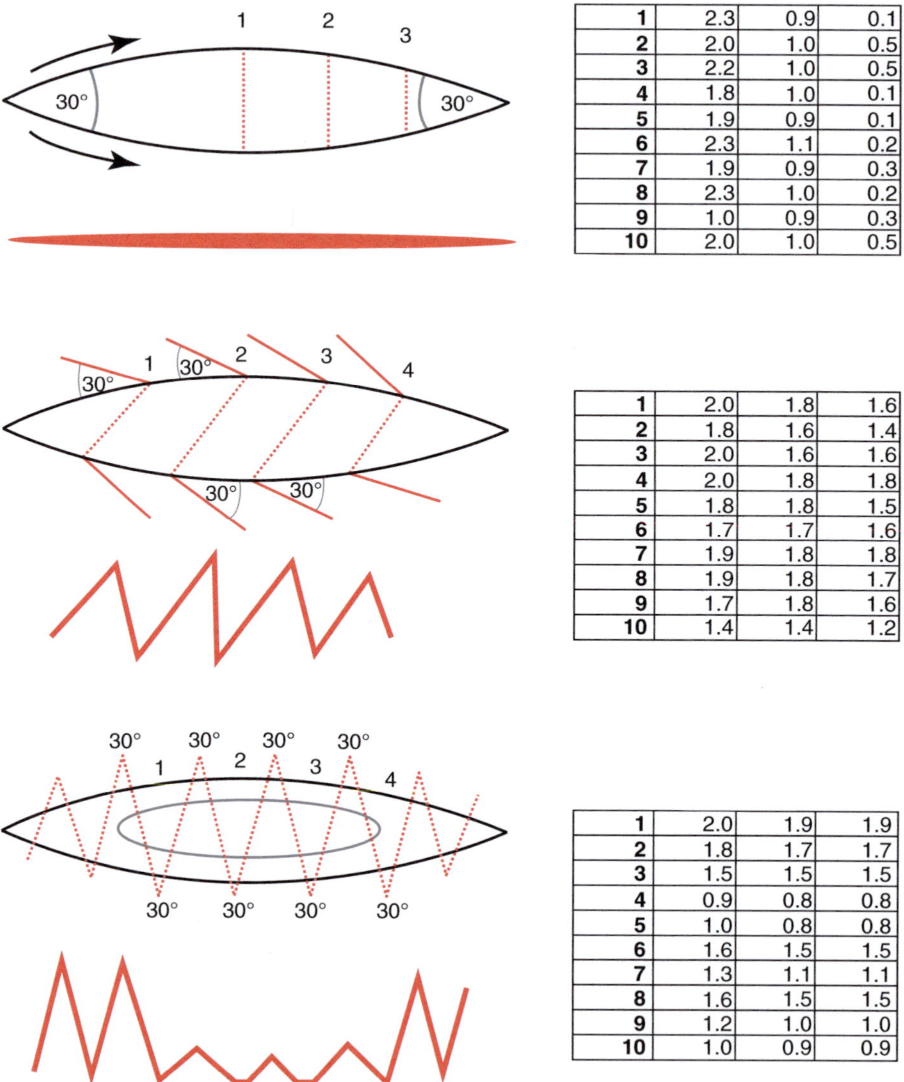

1	2.3	0.9	0.1
2	2.0	1.0	0.5
3	2.2	1.0	0.5
4	1.8	1.0	0.1
5	1.9	0.9	0.1
6	2.3	1.1	0.2
7	1.9	0.9	0.3
8	2.3	1.0	0.2
9	1.0	0.9	0.3
10	2.0	1.0	0.5

1	2.0	1.8	1.6
2	1.8	1.6	1.4
3	2.0	1.6	1.6
4	2.0	1.8	1.8
5	1.8	1.8	1.5
6	1.7	1.7	1.6
7	1.9	1.8	1.8
8	1.9	1.8	1.7
9	1.7	1.8	1.6
10	1.4	1.4	1.2

1	2.0	1.9	1.9
2	1.8	1.7	1.7
3	1.5	1.5	1.5
4	0.9	0.8	0.8
5	1.0	0.8	0.8
6	1.6	1.5	1.5
7	1.3	1.1	1.1
8	1.6	1.5	1.5
9	1.2	1.0	1.0
10	1.0	0.9	0.9

Fig. 7.6 Study comparing wound tension in different closures—simple ellipse, Z-plasty and simple zigzag and points 1, 2 and 3

keeping with already established angle-to-lengthening expectations. The tension measurements were taken prior to closure and summarized in the table.

In the case of the simple elliptical excision, as expected, tension was maximal at the midpoint and very low at the ends. In the case of the simple zigzag, there was a reduction in tension at the midpoint, with a levelling out of forces required to close the wound. In a Z-plasty, there appeared to be more equalization of tension across the wound, however the tension did not lower markedly at the ends of the wound and the midpoint tension was higher than that of a simple zigzag.

Our statistics team applied the Welch's t-test to compare the data between sample groups.

Welch Two Sample t-test comparing data m1 and m2	
t = 1.0989, df = 12.966, p-value = 0.2918	
Alternative hypothesis: true difference in means is not equal to 095% confidence interval:	
−0.1449787	0.4449787
Sample estimates:	
Mean of x	Mean of y
1.97	1.82
Welch Two Sample t-test comparing data: m1 and m3	
t = 3.419, df = 17.953, p-value = 0.003069	
Alternative hypothesis: true difference in means is not equal to 095% confidence interval:	
0.2235329	0.9364671
Sample estimates:	
Mean of x	Mean of y
1.97	1.39
Welch Two Sample t-test comparing data m2 and m3	
t = 3.2819, df = 13.341, p-value = 0.005771	
Alternative hypothesis: true difference in means is not equal to 0	
95% confidence interval:	
0.147679	0.712321
Sample estimates:	
Mean of x	Mean of y
1.82	1.39

The results show clearly that using a simple zigzag reduces tension across the mid-point of the scar more effectively than a Z-plasty (p = 0.005771), and much more effectively than a simple elliptical excision where the tension was highest at the midpoint (p = 0.003069). There was no statistically significant reduction in tension between a Z-plasty and a simple excision (p = 0.2918) in this study.

7.8 Discussion

The techniques of breaking up a scar or incision line by using zigs and zags, in attempts to reduce scarring is not new. However, each of these techniques has specific advantages and disadvantages.

In this study, the Z-plasty did not show a significant reduction of tension when compared to standard elliptical primary closure at the midpoint. This is to be expected as the Z-plasty, by nature of its design, appears to equalize tension across the wound and lengthens the wound. The midpoint scar reduction is a key aim of reducing scarring, especially as authors have shown the link between such tension and scar formation [10].

As this author has noted in a previous article detailing this experiment [52], a simple 30° zigzag not only reduces tension across the wound, <$$$> but also avoids lengthening the scar as much as a Z-plasty. The Z-plasty may be preferable over contractures, but as a primary procedure during excision of a lesion to avoid hypertrophic scarring by reducing wound tension, we found the simple zigzag proved a more effective technique. Given the midpoint is where the lesion to be excised lies, the simple zigzag closure ends up slightly flattened at the midpoint as seen in the clinical photos (Fig. 7.7). In the image pictured the lesion was quite narrow in the horizontal plane, and therefore only two zigzags were possible; however, the wound closed under less tension than would be normally expected and there has been no hypertrophy of the scar. This was a patient who had ended up with keloid or hypertrophic scars on every previous excision on the trunk. At 3 months after surgery she does not have any hypertrophy after the simple zigzag closure (Fig. 7.7).

The study had to be on pigskin so that we could test each pattern on tissue with almost identical characteristics. It would not have been possible to design a clinical study on human patients to compare all the three types of closures on a single patient. However, the study provided valuable insight into the biomechanics of zigs and zags, their role in reducing wound tension, and thereby scarring.

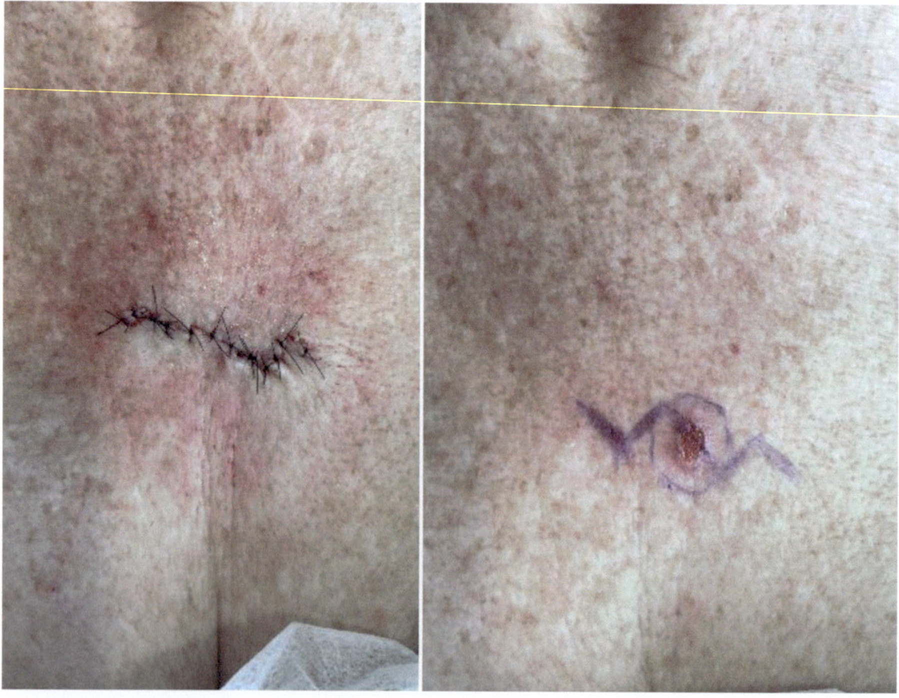

Fig. 7.7 Clinical photo showing zigzag excision to reduce tension

   The author would like to point out an observation that when a 30° angle is used, it functions rather like a Burow's triangle. Burow's triangles, because of the small advancement involved, have been noted to reduce wound tension [53] and this is partly how the simple zigzag works to reduce tension. The zigzag also has the advantage of breaking up the linear scar into many small segments, a method well established in plastic surgical practice to reduce scarring [54].

   As noted previously [52], in a simple elliptical excision, the tension is maximal at the midpoint and tapers off at the ends. Over keloid-prone regions, breaking up scar-lines to reduce tension is helpful. Other surgeons have used "deckled incisions"—sine-wave like irregular incision lines—to break up scar-lines during facial skin lesion excisions, in order to preserve sebaceous glands in areas such as the nose and upper lip where pitted scars occur. Deckling doesn't reduce wound tension [55]. The simple zigzag excision, however, with its 30° angles has this added advantage—and proves an extremely useful option to break up BEST lines in keloid-prone areas, to reduce tension and thereby scar thickness.

References

1. West BR, Applebaum H, Edgerton BW. A better incision for pectus excavatum repair: avoiding the keloid triangle. Pediatr Surg Int. 1994;9:301.
2. Duscher D, Maan ZN, Wong VW, et al. Mechanotransduction and fibrosis. J Biomech. 2014;47(9):1997–2005.
3. Alenghat FJ, Ingber DE. Mechanotransduction: all signals point to cytoskeleton, matrix, and integrins. Sci Signal. 2002;(119):pe6.
4. Gurtner GC, Werner S, Barrandon Y, Longaker MT. Wound repair and regeneration. Nature. 2008;453(7193):314–21.
5. Paul SP. The golden spiral flap: a new flap design that allows for closure of larger wounds under reduced tension—how studying nature's own design led to the development of a new surgical technique. Front Surg. 2016;3:63.
6. Garikipati K. The kinematics of biological growth. Appl Mech Rev. 2009;62(3):030801.
7. Wang Y, Wang N. FRET and mechanobiology. Integr Biol (Camb). 2009;1(10):565–73.
8. Ingber DE. The architecture of life. Sci Am. 1998;278(1):48–57.
9. Aarabi S, Bhatt KA, Shi Y, Paterno J, Chang EI, Loh SA, Holmes JW, Longaker MT, Yee H, Gurtner GC. Mechanical load initiates hypertrophic scar formation through decreased cellular apoptosis. FASEB J. 2007;21(12):3250–61.
10. Gurtner GC, Dauskardt RH, Wong VW, Bhatt KA, Wu K, Vial IN, Padois K, Korman JM, Longaker MT. Improving cutaneous scar formation by controlling the mechanical environment: large animal and phase I studies. Ann Surg. 2011;254(2):217–25.
11. Goto M, Ikeyama K, Tsutsumi M, Denda S, Denda M. Calcium ion propagation in cultured keratinocytes and other cells in skin in response to hydraulic pressure stimulation. J Cell Physiol. 2010;224(1):229–33.
12. Lemmon CA, Chen CS, Romer LH. Cell traction forces direct fibronectin matrix assembly. Biophys J. 2009;96(2):729–38.
13. Deitch EA, Wheelahan TM, Rose MP, Clothier J, Cotter J. Hypertrophic burn scars: analysis of variables. J Trauma. 1983;23:895–8.
14. Akaishi S, Akimoto M, Ogawa R, Hyakusoku H. The relationship between keloid growth pattern and stretching tension: visual analysis using the finite element method. Ann Plast Surg. 2008;60:445–51.

15. Ogawa R, et al. The relationship between skin stretching/contraction and pathologic scarring: the important role of mechanical forces in keloid generation. Wound Repair Regen. 2012;20:149–57.
16. Shockley WW. Scar revision techniques: Z-plasty, W-plasty, and geometric broken line closure. Facial Plast Surg Clin North Am. 2011;19(3):460.
17. Stratton GM. Eye-movements and the aesthetics of visual form. Philos Stud. 1902;20:336–59.
18. Ito H, Yang X. A short line segment squirms along a zigzag line. i-Perception. 2013;4:141–3.
19. Bar M, Neta M. Visual elements of subjective preference modulate amygdala activation. Neuropsychologia. 2006;45:2191–200.
20. Gómez-Puerto G, Munar E, Nadal M. Preference for curvature: a historical and conceptual framework. Front Hum Neurosci. 2016;9:712.
21. Horner WE. Clinical report on the surgical department of the Philadelphia Hospital, Blockley for the months of May, June and July 1837. Am J Med Sci. 1837;21:105–6.
22. Denonvilliers CP. Blepharoplastie. Bull Soc Chir Paris. 1856;7:243–5.
23. Borges AF, Gibson T, et al. The original Z-plasty. Br J Plast Surg. 1973;26(3):237–46.
24. McCurdy SL. Plastic operations to elongate cicatricial contractions across joints. Cleveland Med J. 1904;1:121.
25. Limberg AA. Mathematical principles of local plastic procedures on the surface of the human body. Leningrad: Megriz; 1946.
26. Limberg AA. Design of local flaps. In: Gibson T, editor. Modern trends in plastic surgery, vol. 2. London: Butterworths; 1966.
27. Limberg AA. Skin plastic and shifting triangle flaps in collection of scientific works. Leningrad: Trauma Inst; 1929. p. 862.
28. Limberg AA. Planimetrie und Stereometrie der Hautplastik. Gustav Fischer Verlag: Jena; 1967.
29. Shockley WW. Scar revision techniques: Z-plasty, W-plasty, and geometric broken line closure. Facial Plast Surg Clin North Am. 2011;19(3):455–63.
30. Ellur S, Guido NL. A mathematical model to predict the change in direction of the common limb in Z-plasty. Indian J Plast Surg. 2009;42(1):82–4.
31. Rajabi A, et al. From the rhombic transposition flap toward Z-plasty: an optimized design using the finite element method. J Biomech. 2015;48:3672–8.
32. Borges AF. W-plasty. Ann Plast Surg. 1979;3(2):153–9.
33. Rossoe EWT, Tebcherani AJ, et al. Actinic cheilitis: aesthetic and functional comparative evaluation of vermilionectomy using the classic and W-plasty techniques. An Bras Dermatol. 2011;86(1):65–73.
34. Han S, Han U, et al. W-plasty technique in tracheal reconstruction: a new technique? Eur Surg Res. 2008;41(4):319–23.
35. Beraldo S, Titley G, Allan A. Use of W-plasty in stenotic stoma: a new solution for an old problem. Color Dis. 2006;8(8):715–6.
36. Murakami M, Oki K, et al. The effect of W-plasty on cheek rotation flap. Eplasty. 2010;e8:10.
37. Gómez A, Pomares A. Primary W-plasty closure for surgical repair of the injured lip. J Craniofac Surg. 2016;27(1):e57–8.
38. Elkhatib HA. The extended running W-plasty: an additional tool for simultaneous reduction of the hypertrophied labia minora and redundant clitoral hood. Plast Aesthet Res. 2016;3(11):359–63.
39. Rodgers BA, et al. W-plasty and geometric broken line closure. Facial Plast Surg. 2001;17(4):239–44.
40. Wessberg GA, Hill SC. Revision of facial scars with geometric broken line closure. J Oral Maxillofac Surg. 1982;40(8):492–6.
41. Shockley WW. Scar revision techniques: Z-plasty, W-plasty, and geometric broken line closure. Facial Plast Surg Clin North Am. 2014;22(3):453–62.
42. Elliot D, Cory-Pearce R, Rees GM. The behaviour of presternal scars in a fair-skinned population. Ann R Coll Surg Engl. 1985;67(4):238–40.

43. Meyer M, McGrouther DA. A study relating wound tension to scar morphology in the presternal scar using Langers technique. Br J Plast Surg. 1991;44(4):291.
44. Lanir Y, Fung YC. Two-dimensional mechanical properties of rabbit skin. I. Experimental system. J Biomech. 1974;7(1):29–34.
45. Lanir Y, Fung YC. Two-dimensional mechanical properties of rabbit skin. II. Experimental results. J Biomech. 1974;7(2):171–82.
46. Shockley WW. Scar revision techniques: Z-plasty, W-plasty, and geometric broken line closure. Facial Plast Surg Clin North Am. 2014;22(3):460.
47. Murray JF, Nadel JA. Textbook of respiratory medicine, vol. 1. 2nd ed. Philadelphia: WB Saunders; 1994. p. 531–2.
48. Lang-Lazdunski L, et al. Measurement of chest wall forces on coughing with the use of human cadavers. J Thorac Cardiovasc Surg. 1999;118(6):1157.
49. Ogawa R, et al. The relationship between skin stretching/contraction and pathologic scarring: the important role of mechanical forces in keloid generation. Wound Repair Regen. 2012;20:150–1.
50. Paul SP, et al. A new skin tensiometer device: computational analyses to understand biodynamic excisional skin tension lines. Sci Rep. 2016;6(30117). https://doi.org/10.1038/srep30117.
51. Blinman T. Incisions do not simply sum. Surg Endosc. 2010;24:1746–51. https://doi.org/10.1007/s00464-009-0854-z.
52. Paul SP. The use of zigs and zags to reduce scarring over "Keloid triangles" during excisional surgery: biomechanics, review and recommendations. Surg Sci. 2017;8:240–55.
53. Baker SR. Local flaps in facial reconstruction: expert consult. 3rd ed. Philadelphia: Elsevier Health Sciences; 2014. p. 108.
54. Sharma M, Wakure A. Scar revision. Indian J Plast Surg. 2013;46(2):408–18. https://doi.org/10.4103/0970-0358.118621.
55. Aldred R, Mukherjee P. Deckled incisions in facial surgery. St Vincent's Clin Proc. 2009;17(1):3–7.

Chapter 8
Biodynamic Excisional Skin Tension (BEST) Lines on the Trunk

The tensiometer used in this study has already been discussed in detail [1]. The orientation of the ellipse has been known to be a major determinant of the cosmetic appearance after excisions of a skin lesion, even if there is limited evidence in the literature due to a dearth of clinical studies [2]. We have discussed the pioneering work of Karl Langer in Vienna in studying cleavage lines of skin after creating round clefts and noting the deformations into linear or oval shapes [3]. A retrospective analysis of scars has shown that the final cosmetic outcome can vary depending on the degrees of deviation from these cleavage lines [4].

In this study, the position of each lesion excised was recorded and a map made during the surgical procedure. The skin tensiometer we developed has allowed us to measure pre- and post-tension and map biodynamic excisional skin tension (BEST) lines accurately. A line was marked through the centre of each ellipse and this allowed us to create a body chart of BEST lines for surgical excisions on the trunk and limbs. All excisions were full-thickness skin excisions and the lesions were sent for histopathological examination from whence a record of the dimensions are available. Measurements of the lesions were taken along with a map of the final orientation of closure. BEST lines are important in cutaneous surgery because as many others have suggested—improper incision designs are the main reason for hypertrophic scar responses observed in remodelling wounds [5]. It was also important to map BEST lines across the trunk and upper limbs because wounds which have greater tension on their edges, typically those in the deltoid, upper back and sternal regions have a higher risk of developing excessive scarring [6]. Given this importance of reducing wound tension to reduce scarring, studies have shown that three major components of scar prevention immediately after wound closure are tension relief, hydration and pressure [7]. And adding to the reasons why an accurate guide of BEST lines (lines of least tension) are of great importance to the cutaneous surgeon—recent surveys indicate that 91% of patients who undergo a routine plastic surgical procedure would like improvements to their scars [8].

8.1 Skin Stress and Wound Tension on the Trunk

Skin tension is either due to protrusion of underlying structures and/or the direction of underlying muscle or joints. Wounds therefore gape due to anatomical causes (due to dermal elastin content) or functional causes (joint movements) or physical causes (wound closure under tension) [9]. The concept of Langer's lines or cleavage lines has been established by the observation of ellipsoidal gaping of skin puncture wounds in certain directions.

Prevailing hypotheses suggest that collagen content is greater in one or both directions (horizontal/vertical) depending on repeated stressors, and elastin content may also have a bearing [9]. However, when studies were done by authors on the back region, there was no difference in collagen content suggesting that the skin tension lines and wound tension were not determined by the collagen content of the skin [9]. However, because of daily flexion of the spine during activity, the horizontal direction is expected to handle more stress when compared to the vertical direction and this was borne out in our studies.

On the chest and sternal region, there is no significant difference in the elastin fibre content [9]. However, due to the repeated stretching in the upward and oblique directions due to shoulder movements, the collagen content is greater in the horizontal direction than the vertical direction.

In both the chest, sternal region and back, the pre-dominant direction of BEST lines is in the horizontal direction. However, due to the "rope and razor" effect in the intra-mammary region ("keloid zone"), zigzag incisions have been found to be advisable to reduce tension in this region [10]. In areas such as the sternum, the simple 30° zigzag not only reduces tension across the wound, but also avoids lengthening the scar as much as a traditional Z-plasty does [10].

However, on the lateral chest, the function of respiration causes some changes in biodynamics. Respiration leads to chest expansion, producing maximum stretch in a more vertical direction. The collagen content is significantly also higher in vertical direction than in the horizontal one [9]. This is confirmed by tension studies undertaken that show that in the lateral chest region, BEST lines tend to end up oblique rather than horizontal, as in the case in the scapular region (Fig. 8.1). Overall it is the direction of repeated skin stress that seems to determine the skin's ability to handle tension.

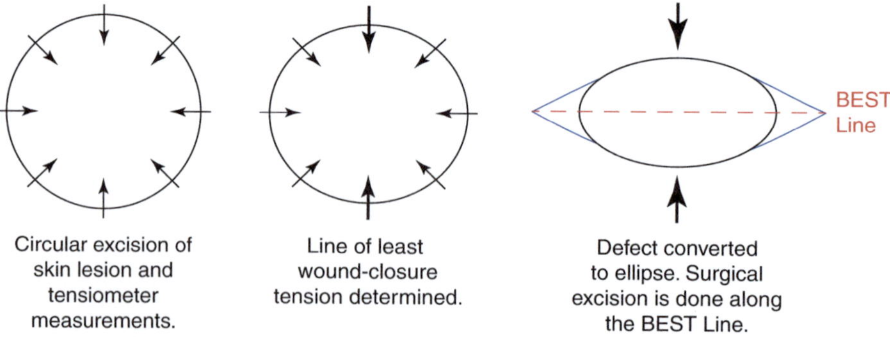

Fig. 8.1 BEST line study methodology

8.2 Superficial Fascial System of the Trunk

Lockwood, who first wrote about the importance of the superficial fascial system (SFS) of the trunk and limbs during plastic surgical procedures considered it an important structure. He felt that repair of the SFS created a more stable scar that healed without migration and therefore caused less gaping of wounds [11]. Others have suggested that the repair of the superficial fascial system (SFS) basically caused a reduction of tension on skin flaps, and provide longer-lasting support to the wound bed [12]. Many authors have written that closing the superficial fascial system on the back and limbs reduced the dead space and therefore seroma formation [12]. Indeed, this was the prevailing view and standard teaching during this author's plastic surgical training.

The ability of skin and fluid to "creep" has been exploited in plastic surgery for wound closures, especially while using tissue expanders [13], and during burn management [14]. Essentially this mechanical creep is due to the viscoelastic properties of skin; creep and stress relaxation allow skin to stretch beyond its normal state within a short period of time [15].

A significant study into the properties of the superficial fascial system was undertaken by Song and Askari [16]. While Lockwood had noted reduction in wound-width [11], there had been no conclusive scientific evidence that repair of the superficial fascial layer increased the biomechanical strength of surgical wounds. This study [16] looked to assess both early postoperative and long-term wound strength following closure of the superficial fascial system of the trunk. The authors noted that repair of the superficial fascial system transfers tension from the dermis to deeper tissues, minimizing tension to skin flaps of the wound. The biomechanical properties of this energy transfer was amplified by the dermis-superficial fascia junctional architecture—wherein the continuity of the dermis to the fascia ensures direct energy transfer, while the obliquely and vertically oriented fascial septae are found to disperse energy in a direction perpendicular to the wound tension [16]. In an *ex vivo* study, repair of superficial fascial system in addition to the dermis had a major impact on wound tensile strength. Studies on the superficial fascial system show that it can handle rigorous biomechanical testing on its own, indicating that fascia has its own viscoelastic response pattern to stress [17].

Song and Askari made the following conclusions [16]:

1. The direct continuity of the dermal-superficial fascial junction and the nearly identical connective tissue content make the SFS an extension of the dermis.
2. When the superficial fascial system (SFS) is incorporated into surgical repair, it enhances the initial biomechanical strength, while effectively closing the dead space. This technique is therefore of great use on the trunk and limbs especially.
3. Closure of the superficial fascial system (SFS) can be expected to decrease the incidence of mechanical wound dehiscence compared to dermal sutures alone.

What this means that the superficial fascial system is a dynamic viscoelastic layer and not a passive scaffold for subcutaneous fat. The fascia maintains body contours and it is therefore especially important that the superficial fascial system is closed with sutures during body contouring procedures. Conceptually, this author considers that the superficial fascial system is not dissimilar to the superficial musculo-aponeurotic system (SMAS) of the face. And just as plication of the SMAS is used in facelifts, in excisional wounds after large skin cancers or lesions, it is especially important that the superficial fascial system (SFS) of the trunk and limbs is not ignored. This practice confers both a biomechanical advantage and also closes the dead space, thereby reducing the risk of seroma formation.

8.3 BEST Lines on the Trunk and Limbs

The tensiometer used for this study has been described previously [1] and the statistical validity of the technique has already been published in previous papers [18, 19]. The initial study of BEST lines conducted on the scalp showed that closing using BEST lines (which run in a coronal direction on the scalp) showed a clear advantage. The coronal (BEST line) tension on the scalp was noted to be significantly different (less) when compared with both the sagittal and oblique skin tension measurements (two-sided paired t-test, unequal variances; $p = 0.00075$ and 0.000013 respectively) [19].

This research was conducted in the context of a PhD study undertaken by this author investigating BEST lines across the body. Results of facial lesions will be discussed separately in another chapter. Ethics approvals [New Zealand: Health and Disability Ethics Committee (HDEC Reference number 15/CEN/113); Australia: University of Queensland Institutional Human Ethics (Approval No. 2015001550)] were obtained from the relevant authorities. This study was carried out in accordance with the recommendations of the ethics committees listed above, with written informed consent from all subjects. All subjects gave written informed consent in accordance with the Declaration of Helsinki.

One thousand one hundred and eighty one (1181) consecutive skin lesion excisions (Table 8.1) were examined (age range 13–95; median age 64). The clear majority were for skin cancer and the others were for cysts or dysplastic naevi. Lesions such as lipomata, which entail incisional rather than excisional surgery i.e. where overlying skin was not excised were excluded from this study. All lesions were cut out in a circular fashion (Fig. 8.1) and any pre-tension of skin was noted. It was generally noted that shoulder and scapular movements result in significant ventral and dorsal pre-tension which can give rise to erroneous calculations of skin tension using the pinch method of determining RSTL, leading to wounds being closed under greater tension. The tensiometer was used to determine line of least tension and a map was made of BEST lines across the human body (Figs. 8.2 and 8.3). The lesion dimensions were measured (Table 8.2) at the pathology lab after tissue

Table 8.1 Site and numbers of excisions included in this study

Body site of excision	Number of lesions
Trunk (chest/abdomen/back/groin)	376
Upper limb (arm/forearm/hand)	168
Lower limb (arm/forearm/hand)	166
Head and Neck (scalp/upper back)	471

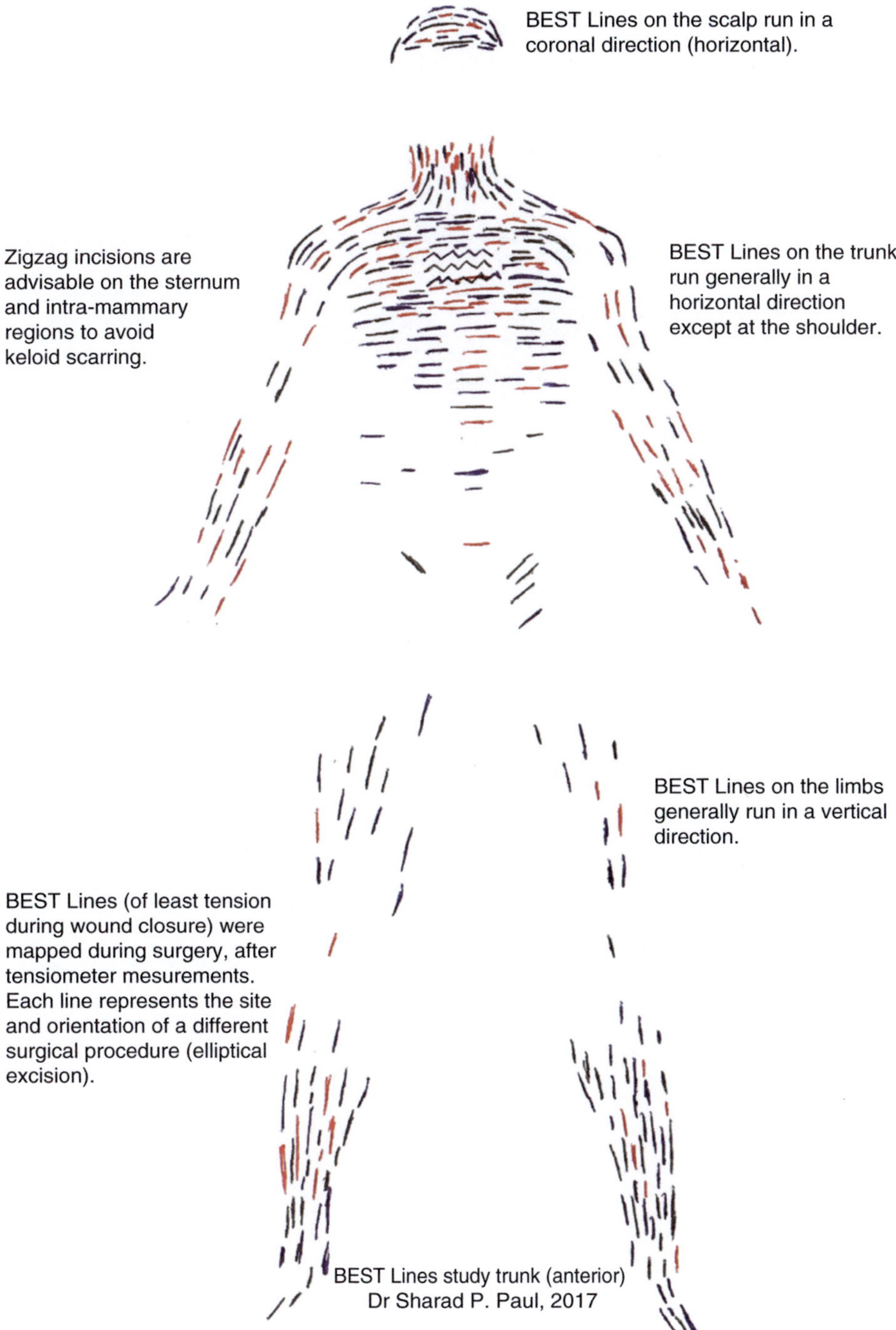

Fig. 8.2 BEST line study—each line represents the orientation of closure of a different surgical excision

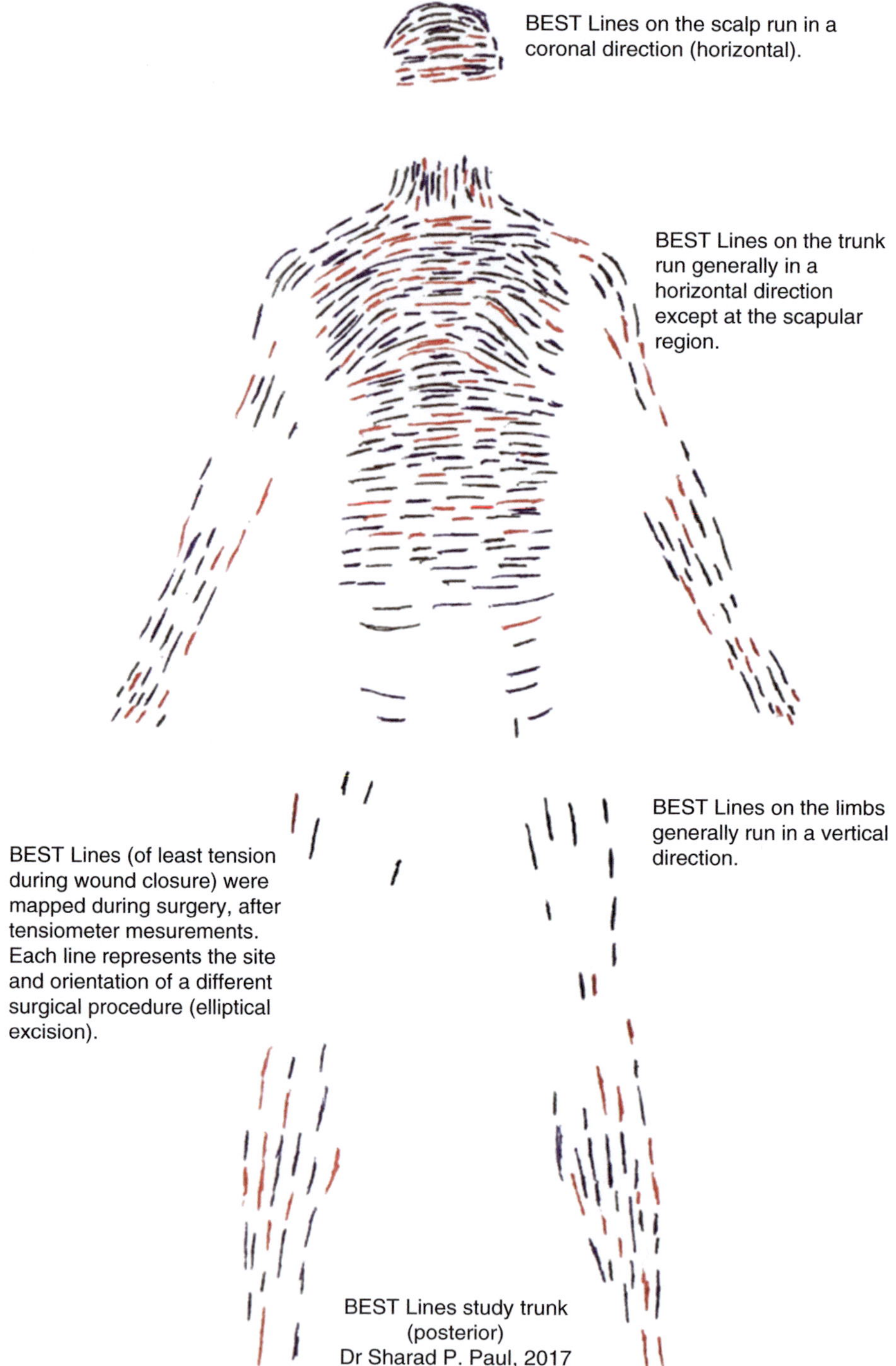

Fig. 8.3 BEST line study—each line represents the orientation of closure of a different surgical excision

Table 8.2 BEST line study excisions

No	Age	Sex	Region	Diameter (cm)	Location
1	88	F	L limb	2.5	R ankle
2	88	F	L limb	1.5	R thigh
3	82	M	Face	3.2	R zygomatic region
4	61	F	Trunk	3.2	Mid back
5	71	M	Face	1	L temple
6	71	M	Trunk	1	L back
7	71	M	Face	0.4	L eyelid
8	95	M	Ear	1.8	R ear
9	69	M	Trunk	2.7	R back
10	69	M	U limb	0.8	L hand
11	69	M	U limb	1.2	R forearm
12	82	F	U limb	4.5	L arm
13	82	F	U limb	2.5	R arm
14	82	F	l limb	0.4	R calf
15	65	M	U limb	1.6	R hand
16	65	M	U limb	1.3	R calf
17	63	M	Trunk	0.5	Abdominal wall
18	67	F	Trunk	3	Mid back
19	41	F	Trunk	0.5	Chest
20	78	M	U limb	1.8	L forearm
21	38	F	L limb	0.6	L foot
22	83	F	L limb	3.7	L leg/ankle
23	16	M	Lip	0.3	Upper lip
24	64	M	U limb	0.4	L ring finger
25	67	M	U limb	0.9	R shoulder
26	55	M	Trunk	0.6	L buttock
27	81	F	L limb	3.3	L leg
28	84	M	Face	2	R temple
29	79	F	L limb	2	R foot
30	60	M	Face	3.5	R cheek
31	67	M	Trunk	2.4	R scapular
32	56	F	Trunk	0.7	R lower back
33	74	M	Trunk	3.2	Mid back
34	35	F	Trunk	0.4	L upper back
35	55	F	Lip	0.3	Upper lip
36	55	F	L limb	0.5	R thigh
37	62	F		2	Scalp
38	32	F	L limb	0.9	L upper thigh
39	73	F	U limb	1	L hand
40	75	F	L limb	2.3	L foot
41	75	F	L limb	1.3	R thigh

(continued)

Table 8.2 (continued)

No	Age	Sex	Region	Diameter (cm)	Location
42	64	F	Face	3	R cheek
43	73	M	L limb	4	R leg anterior
44	73	M	L limb	3.4	R calf
45	83	M	Face	1.3	L nose cheek
46	83	M	Face	1.6	L nose
47	83	M	L limb	0.6	R leg anterior
48	71	M	Trunk	2.2	Lower back
49	81	F	Face	0.9	R lower eyelid
50	71	F	Face	0.7	Anterior neck
51	60	F	Face	1.7	L lower eyelid
52	64	M	U limb	2.1	R forearm
53	74	F	Face	1.2	L neck trapezius
54	66	F	L limb	2	L thigh
55	38	F	Face	1.2	R forehead
56	68	F	U limb	2.7	L hand wrist
57	77	M	U limb	2.1	L forearm
58	68	M	Face	1	Posterior neck back
59	38	M	Trunk	3.4	Mid back
60	38	M	Face	0.5	R ear
61	76	F	L limb	0.6	L foot
62	76	F	L limb	1.1	R leg anterior
63	72	M	Trunk	0.6	L back
64	59	F	Trunk	1.5	R back
65	68	F	Trunk	3.3	R flank
66	52	M	Face	1.2	L ear
67	80	M	Trunk	0.7	R back
68	70	M	Trunk	3.3	R shoulder
69	70	M	Face	1.4	R pre-auricular
70	64	M	Face	1.3	Upper neck
71	64	M	Face	1.8	Lower neck
72	57	M	Ear	0.4	L ear
73	63	F	U limb	0.7	L shoulder
74	67	F	U limb	1.6	L hand
75	34	M	Trunk	0.7	L chest
76	79	F	L limb	0.4	R ankle
77	20	M	Face	0.7	Forehead
78	54	F	U limb	1.8	L shoulder
79	57	M	L limb	1.1	R sole foot
80	57	F	Trunk	2	L breast
81	69	M	L limb	2.4	R leg lateral
82	74	M	L limb	1.4	R thigh

Table 8.2 (continued)

No	Age	Sex	Region	Diameter (cm)	Location
83	69	M	Trunk	2.2	L back
84	43	F	Trunk	1.1	R upper back
85	90	F	U limb	1.5	R wrist
86	90	F	L limb	2.1	L foot dorsum
87	59	F	Trunk	1.2	R breast
88	80	M	L limb	3	L leg
89	74	M	Scalp	0.5	Scalp
90	52	F	Face	0.4	L temple
91	52	F	Trunk	0.4	L trapezius
92	33	M	Face	2.4	L temple
93	51	M	Scalp	0.4	Scalp
94	27	M	Face	0.4	Face L cheek
95	51	F	Face	1.5	L neck
96	63	M	Face	0.8	Forehead
97	63	M	L limb	1.2	R thigh
98	88	M	Face	2.4	Scalp
99	72	M	Trunk	0.9	L chest
100	70	F	Face	0.7	L cheek
101	56	M	Trunk	2.2	Chest
102	56	M	Trunk	2	Abdominal wall
103	65	F	Trunk	0.9	Upper back
104	76	M	Face	1.6	L cheek
105	78	F	L limb	2.5	R thigh
106	66	M	U limb	3	R forearm
107	36	F	Trunk	0.4	L axillary
108	72	M	Face	0.4	R ear
109	68	F	Trunk	3	L chest
110	38	M	Trunk	0.9	Upper back
111	81	M	U limb	1.5	L arm
112	73	F	Scalp	0.7	Scalp
114	50	F	Scalp	2	Scalp
115	58	M	Face	1	R cheek
116	61	M	Face	0.4	Lower lip
117	51	F	Face	1	L nose
118	70	M	Face	1.8	R temple
119	83	M	Trunk	1	R groin
120	74	M	Face	1.5	L neck
121	74	M	Face	1.5	L cheek
122	74	M	Face	0.6	Forehead
123	45	F	U limb	0.4	R forearm
124	82	F	U limb	2	L forearm
125	70	M	Scalp	2	R scalp

(continued)

Table 8.2 (continued)

No	Age	Sex	Region	Diameter (cm)	Location
126	78	M	Face	1.3	R pre-auricular
127	62	M	Trunk	1.3	Back
128	77	M	U limb	0.6	L forearm
129	81	M	L limb	0.5	R leg
130	81	M	L Limb	0.4	L leg
131	45	M	Face	1.7	L ear posterior
132	42	M	Trunk	1.3	L back
133	67	F	L limb	2.9	L leg medial
134	67	F	L limb	1.4	L leg lateral
135	58	M	Face	1.1	Neck posterior
136	49	F	L limb	0.4	L thigh
137	79	F	Face	2	R eyebrow
138	27	F	L limb	0.4	L thigh
139	83	F	L limb	3.4	R leg ankle
140	60	F	U limb	2	R forearm
141	40	M	Trunk	1.1	L chest
142	55	F	U limb	0.8	L arm
143	55	F	Trunk	0	L lower abdomen
144	74	M	Trunk	2.1	L back
145	51	M	Trunk	1.6	L back
146	42	F	Trunk	2	L back
147	41	F	Face	0.5	R cheek
148	41	F	Face	0.6	L neck
149	62	F	Face	0.8	R cheek
150	72	M	Face	0.9	R temple
151	72	M	Trunk	1.7	R chest
152	76	F	Trunk	3	Back
153	73	M	Trunk	2	Back
154	81	F	Trunk	1.8	Chest
155	80	M	Trunk	4.2	R scapular
156	80	M	U limb	1.6	R arm
157	88	F	L limb	1.6	R thigh posterior
158	88	F	L limb	1.4	R thigh lower
159	61	M	Face	1.5	L forehead
160	65	M	Face	1	R cheek lateral
161	65	M	Face	0.5	R cheek medial
162	66	M	U limb	2.2	R forearm
163	84	M	Face	3.4	L cheek
164	26	M	Face	0.4	Lower lip
165	59	M	L limb	0.8	R leg
166	59	M	L limb	1.8	R ankle

Table 8.2 (continued)

No	Age	Sex	Region	Diameter (cm)	Location
167	49	F	L limb	2	L leg
168	62	F	U limb	1.4	L hand
169	59	M	Neck	2.5	L neck
170	75	F	Trunk	1.6	Back
171	75	F	Neck	0.7	Neck posterior
172	41	F	Face	0.4	L cheek
173	55	F	Trunk	0.9	Upper back
174	71	M	Trunk	0.7	L groin
175	83	F	U limb	2.5	R forearm
176	83	F	U Limb	2.4	L arm
177	83	F	Trunk	3.2	L scapular
178	57	M	Neck	2	Neck
179	76	F	L limb	0.7	L thigh posterior
180	64	F	Face	4.5	R cheek
181	37	M	Trunk	0.4	Chest
182	61	M	L limb	1.8	L knee
183	48	M	Face	1.7	Anterior nose
184	75	M	Trunk	2.3	Mid upper back
185	58	F	Trunk	0.8	Back
186	58	F	U limb	0.7	R arm
187	58	M	U limb	1	R forearm
188	83	M	Trunk	0.9	Mid upper back
189	45	F	L limb	1.8	L leg medial
190	64	F	Trunk	0.9	Chest
191	64	F	L limb	0.7	L thigh
192	67	F	Face	1.2	Forehead
193	64	M	Face	1.2	L ear posterior
194	85	F	L limb	1.6	L leg
195	63	F	L limb	1	L calf
196	43	F	Trunk	1	Back
197	43	F	Face	0.4	R cheek
198	44	F	Trunk	2.5	Upper back
199	81	F	Neck	1.7	L neck
200	52	F	L limb	1	L leg
201	80	M	Face	0.5	R temple
202	64	F	U limb	1.2	L hand
203	85	F	Face	2.2	R cheek
204	60	M	L limb	1.2	R leg anterior
205	83	F	U limb	2.5	R arm
206	83	F	L limb	1.5	R leg
207	83	F	U limb	3.5	R hand
208	68	F	Trunk	1	Chest

(continued)

Table 8.2 (continued)

No	Age	Sex	Region	Diameter (cm)	Location
209	75	M	U limb	3.2	L forearm
210	75	M	Trunk	2.5	R chest
211	87	M	Trunk	1.8	Groin
212	61	M	Scalp	1.8	Scalp
213	69	F	Trunk	2	R back
214	69	F	Face	0.6	L neck
215	66	M	Trunk	1	R back
216	46	F	Trunk	2	L back
217	64	F	Trunk	1.5	Back
218	74	M	Trunk	0.8	R mid back
219	78	M	Face	2.6	R cheek
220	20	M	Face	1	Chin
221	74	F	Trunk	3.7	R neck
222	69	M	Trunk	3.5	Mid upper back
223	54	M	Face	2	Neck posterior
224	54	M	Face	0.7	R neck
225	70	F	Face	1.2	L cheek
226	95	F	Face	2.4	L eyebrow
227	95	F	Scalp	1.3	Scalp
228	85	F	L Limb	3.8	L leg
229	58	M	Scalp	2.5	Scalp
230	41	M	Face	0.7	R cheek
231	60	M	Trunk	2.6	Chest
232	54	M	Face	3.6	L temple
233	54	M	Ear	1.3	R ear
234	77	M	Lower limb	5	L leg
235	77	M	Trunk	3.5	Upper back
236	39	F	Trunk	1.5	upper back
237	66	F	L limb	1	R thigh
238	66	F	L limb	0.6	R calf
239	76	F	Trunk	4.5	R upper back
240	76	F	L limb	1.2	R foot
241	66	M	U limb	2.5	R forearm
242	62	M	Face	0.9	L cheek
243	62	M	Face	0.6	L ear posterior
244	88	F	Trunk	1.5	R ankle
245	88	F	Trunk	2	R back
246	79	F	L limb	1	L foot dorsum
247	79	F	L limb	2	L leg pretibial
248	50	M	Trunk	1.7	L upper back
249	68	F	U limb	1	L arm
250	74	M	L limb	4	L leg

Table 8.2 (continued)

No	Age	Sex	Region	Diameter (cm)	Location
251	70	M	Face	0.8	L cheek
252	54	M	Trunk	0.8	L scapular
253	55	F	U limb	1	R hand
254	72	M	Trunk	3.7	Mid back
255	67	F	Trunk	1	L scapular
256	74	M	U limb	1.8	R hand
257	64	F	Trunk	0.9	Chest
258	72	M	L limb	2.1	R leg
259	72	M	L limb	1.5	L leg
260	71	M	L limb	3	R lower leg
261	58	M	L limb	2.5	L calf
262	72	M	Ear	3	R post auricular
263	56	M	Trunk	0.8	Upper back
264	56	M	Trunk	0.6	L buttock
265	61	F	Trunk	2.5	L upper back
266	54	M	Trunk	0.5	Upper back
267	79	M	Face	0.8	R cheek
268	69	F	L limb	0.9	L groin
269	33	M	Face	1	Neck posterior
270	73	F	Trunk	2.2	Back
271	46	F	Face	0.8	L eyelid
272	67	M	Trunk	4.1	R back
273	75	M	Trunk	1.6	Back
274	77	M	Face	1.5	R mandibular
275	77	M	Face	1.8	R pre-auricular
276	72	M	Trunk	0.7	L axillary
277	34	M	Trunk	0.7	Chest
278	61	M	Face	2.5	R cheek
279	65	F	Face	1.5	R nose
280	87	M	Face	1.2	R inner canthus
281	75	M	Face	1.7	R neck
282	61	M	Face	1.8	R ear post-auricular
283	73	F	Trunk	0.5	L breast
284	47	F	Trunk	0.6	R shoulder
285	62	F	Trunk	1.5	R flank
286	62	M	Trunk	0.4	Abdominal wall
287	76	M	Face	0.5	Forehead
288	65	M	Face	3	R scalp
289	63	M	Face	3.5	Scalp vertex
290	40	F	Face	1.4	L temple
291	40	F	Face	0.8	Upper back

(continued)

Table 8.2 (continued)

No	Age	Sex	Region	Diameter (cm)	Location
292	70	M	Trunk	2	L back
293	84	M	Ear	2	L ear
294	43	F	Trunk	4.5	Mid back
295	68	M	L limb	3.5	R leg lower
296	68	M	L limb	3.5	R leg upper
297	68	M	L limb	4.5	L leg lateral
298	68	M	Face	2	Scalp
299	70	M	Face	4.5	L forehead
300	34	F	U limb	2.2	R forearm
301	34	F	U limb	2.6	L forearm
302	70	F	L limb	0.8	L leg
303	73	F	L limb	2	L leg
304	63	F	Face	0.8	R cheek
305	63	M	Face	2	R ear
306	61	M	Trunk	0.5	Chest central
307	90	F	Face	1	R ear
308	81	M	Face	1.4	R lower eyelid
309	81	M	Face	0.4	Neck posterior
310	72	M	Trunk	1.3	R lower leg
311	36	F	Face	1.1	L cheek
312	34	F	Trunk	0.5	Abdominal wall
313	34	F	Face	0.5	L neck
314	92	M	L limb	1	L foot dorsum
315	92	M	L limb	0.8	R leg
316	50	F	Trunk	1	Mid back
317	59	M	U limb	1	L forearm
318	70	M	Face	2.2	Scalp
319	37	F	Face	0.4	Chin
320	75	F	Trunk	2	L shoulder upper
321	75	F	Trunk	2	L shoulder lower
322	78	F	L limb	2.2	R calf
323	59	M	Trunk	2.5	R upper back
324	70	M	Trunk	1.5	L upper back
325	13	M	Scalp	0.9	L scalp
326	80	M	L limb	4	L calf
327	80	M	Face	2.5	R neck
328	58	F	Face	1.8	L neck
329	55	F	Face	1.3	Forehead
330	55	F	Face	1.4	L cheek
331	80	M	Face	0.9	L cheek
332	65	F	Trunk	1.7	Chest wall
333	65	F	Face	0.5	R cheek

Table 8.2 (continued)

No	Age	Sex	Region	Diameter (cm)	Location
334	71	F	Face	0.5	R neck
335	80	F	L limb	3	L leg pretibial
336	80	F	Nose	1.5	Nose bridge
337	78	F	L limb	0.4	R calf
338	69	F	Nose	0.8	Anterior nose
339	63	M	Trunk	2	R back
340	63	M	Trunk	0.7	Back midline
341	73	M	U limb	4.3	L wrist
342	73	M	Trunk	2.4	Mid back
343	73	M	U limb	3	R elbow
344	49	M	Face	1.2	L cheek
345	84	F	Face	2	Forehead
346	84	F	L limb	0.8	L leg
347	84	F	L limb	0.5	R thigh
348	80	M	L limb	2.3	L leg upper
349	80	M	L limb	2.4	L leg lower
350	77	M	U limb	3.2	R forearm
351	80	M	Face	1	L neck
352	71	F	Face	1.7	R cheek
353	57	M	Face	0.7	R temple
354	80	M	Scalp	3.2	Scalp vertex
355	90	F	Trunk	4.5	Back lower
356	60	M	U limb	3.8	L forearm
357	31	F	L limb	1.1	R thigh
358	76	M	L limb	4.5	R leg
359	76	F	Trunk	1.2	L breast
360	54	F	U limb	1.7	R hand
361	54	F	U limb	1.4	L hand
362	74	M	U limb	2.8	L hand
363	74	M	U limb	2.1	L wrist
364	74	M	Face	2.1	R neck
365	74	M	Trunk	2.9	R scapular
366	84	M	Face	1	Scalp
367	84	M	U limb	0.8	L forearm
368	51	F	U limb	1	R forearm
369	66	F	U limb	0.5	L hand
370	85	F	Face	1.5	Nose bridge
371	85	F	L limb	2	L leg pretibial
372	85	F	L limb	0.8	L leg lateral
373	84	F	U limb	2	R hand dorsum
374	83	M	Trunk	4.1	L axillary back
375	65	M	Trunk	0.6	Lower back

(continued)

Table 8.2 (continued)

No	Age	Sex	Region	Diameter (cm)	Location
376	65	M	Trunk	0.7	Upper back
377	93	F	Face	3	R forehead
378	81	F	Face	2.2	L cheek
379	48	F	U limb	0.6	L arm upper
380	76	M	L limb	0.6	R leg lower
381	61	M	Face	0.5	R neck
382	44	F	L limb	0.5	R leg
383	85	F	Face	0.8	R neck
384	85	F	Trunk	0.6	L abdominal wall
385	36	F	Face	0.5	L cheek
386	36	F	Face	0.6	R cheek
387	60	M	U limb	2.1	R forearm
388	77		Neck	1.4	Neck posterior
389			Trunk	1.4	L breast
390	62	F	L limb	1.2	L calf
391	44	F	Face	0.5	R cheek
392	86	M	Ear	1.5	R ear
393	78	F	L limb	3.5	R leg
394	78	F	U limb	2.3	L forearm
395	58	M	Trunk	3.1	L lower back
396	42	F	Face	1.4	Forehead
397	69	F	L limb	2.5	R tendo-Achilles
398	65	F	Face	2	R neck
399	78	F	Face	1.8	L arm
400	53	F	Face	1.7	L cheek
401	77	F	L limb	1.2	L leg
402	77	F	L limb	1.7	L tendo-Achilles calf
403	52	F	Trunk	1.7	R clavicular
404	57	F	U limb	0.6	L forearm
405	45	F	Face	0.8	R cheek
406	67	M	Trunk	2	R chest
407	62	F	U limb	1.6	R forearm
408	62	F	U limb	1	L hand
409	62	F	U limb	0.6	L forearm
410	73	M	Ear	1	R ear
411	73	M	Trunk	2.1	Chest sternum
412	62	F	L limb	1.8	L calf
413	87	M	Trunk	3	Back
414	73	F	Face	1.6	R neck
415	20	F	Face	0.6	Neck posterior

Table 8.2 (continued)

No	Age	Sex	Region	Diameter (cm)	Location
416	82	F	Trunk	2	L scapular
417	84	M	Trunk	1.5	R chest
418	84	M	Trunk	0.5	R lower back
419	86	F	Face	2	R temple
420	86	F	Face	1.6	L cheek
421	79	F	L limb	2.7	L ankle foot
422	44	F	Trunk	0.5	R foot
423	83	F	L limb	1.8	R leg
424	37	F	U limb	3.4	L shoulder
425	37	M	U limb	0.6	L forearm
426	73	M	Face	0.4	R ear
427	58	F	Face	0.7	L forehead
428	80	M	L limb	3.2	R pretibial
429	65	F	U limb	1.7	R arm
430	69	M	U limb	2	R arm
431	87	M	Trunk	2.2	Upper back
432	37	F	Trunk	0.8	Upper back
433	64	M	Trunk	2	L clavicular
434	50	F	L limb	0.7	L Leg
435	75	M	Face	0.3	Eyelid
436	49	M	Face	0.4	Neck posterior
437	49	M	Face	0.9	R ear
438	64	F	U limb	2.3	R arm
439	54	F	U limb	4	L forearm
440	60	F	Trunk	2	L scapular
441	48	F	Trunk	0.5	R chest
442	73	M	U limb	2.3	R forearm
443	73	M	U limb	2	R hand
444	68	F	L limb	0.9	R posterior thigh
445	68	M	L Limb	1.2	R popliteal fossa
446	86	F	Face	0.7	L cheek
447	65	M	L limb	1.8	R leg
448	80	M	Face	0.7	L neck
449	36	F	Face	0.4	R cheek
450	36	M	Trunk	0.7	Chest
451	63	M	Face	2.6	R temple
452	50	M	Trunk	2	R chest
453	50	M	Trunk	1.8	L back
454	50	M	Trunk	3.5	R back
455	86	F	U limb	3	L arm
456	76	M	U limb	2.8	R forearm
457	54	M	Face	0.5	L neck

(continued)

Table 8.2 (continued)

No	Age	Sex	Region	Diameter (cm)	Location
458	54	M	Face	1.2	L eyelid
459	57	M	L limb	3	R pretibial
460	72	M	Scalp	3	Occipital scalp
461	72	M	Face	0.5	L nose
462	54	M	Scalp	1.4	R scalp
463	59	M	Face	2.2	Forehead
464	60	F	U limb	1.7	R forearm
465	17	F	Lip	0.3	Lower lip
466	81	F	L limb	3.5	L leg
467	56	F	Neck	0.5	R neck
468	56	F	Trunk	0.4	Upper back
469	82	F	Nose	0.9	L nose
470	74	M	Face	1.9	Forehead
471	38	M	L limb	0.5	R calf
472	81	M	L limb	3	R calf
473	33	F	U limb	0.7	L forearm
474	69	F	Face	0.3	L cheek
475	61	F	Face	0.6	R ala nasi
476	90	M	Face	1.8	R ear
477	80	M	Trunk	4.2	L clavicular
478	56	F	Neck	2	R neck
479	69	M	Trunk	4	Mid back
480	43	F	Face	2.4	R neck
481	56	M	Trunk	1.7	L back
482	63	F	Trunk	2.5	R back
483	73	M	Face	1	R nose
484	74	M	Face	2	Anterior neck
485	58	F	Face	1.2	R cheek
486	49	F	Trunk	0.5	R breast
487	49	F	Trunk	0.5	R back
488	77	F	Face	1.2	Nose bridge
489	77	F	Face	1.8	R cheek
490	78	M	Trunk	1	L scapular
491	52	F	Trunk	3	R buttock
492	53	F	U limb	2.5	L forearm
493	47	M	Face	1.7	Nasal tip
494	51	F	Lip	1	Upper lip
495	51	F	Trunk	0.7	Left scapular
496	45	F	Face	0.3	R ala nasi
497	67	F	Face	0.4	L temple
498	68	M	Scalp	2.3	R mastoid
499	69	F	U limb	2	L upper triceps

Table 8.2 (continued)

No	Age	Sex	Region	Diameter (cm)	Location
500	39	F	Trunk	1.2	R back
501	39	F	Trunk	0.8	Abdomen
502	75	F	U limb	2	R hand
503	68	F	Face	0.5	Nasal tip
504	56	M	L limb	1.7	L lower leg
505	51	M	Trunk	0.8	L scapular
506	83	M	Trunk	3.5	Anterior chest
507	46	M	L limb	0.7	L leg lateral
508	41	F	Trunk	0.9	Abdomen
509	69	F	L limb	4	L knee
510	77	M	Face	0.7	L scalp
511	78	M	Ear	2.1	L posterior helix
512	44	F	Trunk	1.7	R scapular
513	46	F	L limb	1	L thigh
514	46	F	Face	0.7	L cheek
515	76	M	Face	2	L temple
516	76	M	Ear	0.7	Infra-auricular
517	75	F	Face	0.6	Forehead
518	69	F	U limb	2	L forearm
519	34	F	Trunk	3	L shoulder
520	55	F	U limb	3	R shoulder
521	71	F	Trunk	4.2	Upper back
522	71	F	Trunk	3	Upper back
523	63	M	Face	1.7	R temple
524	62	F	L limb	2	L leg
525	80	F	Face	1.2	Anterior nose
526	76	F	L limb	3.7	R leg
527	62	F	L limb	2.7	Popliteal fossa
528	86	M	Face	1.8	R ear
529	65	F	Face	1.1	L cheek
530	74	M	L limb	2.5	L calf
531	74	M	Face	0.7	L neck
532	72	F	Trunk	0.4	Chest
533	49	F	U limb	0.8	L hand
534	49	F	Face	0.3	L neck
535	73	F	Trunk	1.3	R chest
536	72	M	L limb	2.4	L lateral leg
537	70	F	Trunk	4.5	L sternal region
538	80	M	L limb	1.6	R thigh
539	80	M	L limb	3.7	R leg
540	67	M	Trunk	0.7	L lower back
541	74	F	Face	4	R neck

(continued)

Table 8.2 (continued)

No	Age	Sex	Region	Diameter (cm)	Location
542	64	M	Neck	1	L neck
543	83	M	L limb	1.8	Pre-tibial
544	83	M	Trunk	1.4	Chest wall
545	83	M	Face	1	L ear
546	75	M	L limb	2.5	L thigh
547	69	F	U limb	2	Forearm
548	19	M	Scalp	0.5	Scalp
549	17	F	U limb	1.2	L wrist
550	11	F	Face	0.4	Forehead
551	62	M	Trunk	1.2	R back
552	35	M	Face	4	Forehead
553	79	M	L limb	2.5	R leg
554	79	M	U limb	1.6	L forearm
555	69	M	U limb	3.5	R forearm
556	71	F	Face	1.3	Nasal tip
557	90	M	L limb	1.6	R knee
558	87	F	U limb	1.8	R forearm
559	70	F	U limb	2.2	L hand
560	78	M	L limb	0.9	R calf
561	53	M	Lip	2	Lower lip
562	53	M	Trunk	0.7	Back
563	70	F	Nose	0.5	ala nasi
564	69	M	Face	1.4	L ear
565	53	F	Face	0.8	Anterior neck
566	88	M	Face	2.5	Posterior scalp
567	88	M	Face	1.8	Left scalp
568	54	F	Trunk	1.2	Chest
569	84	F	Trunk	3.6	Upper back
570	64	F	Trunk	1.4	Upper back
571	64	F	U limb	0.9	Left hand
572	62	F	Face	2.2	R cheek
573	87	F	Face	0.7	Lower lip
574	67	F	U limb	2	R hand
575	77	F	Face	0.7	Left cheek
576	74	M	Face	3.5	Posterior scalp
577	46	F	Face	1.3	Right eyelid
578	64	M	U limb	2	R wrist
579	64	M	U limb	0.5	R hand
580	90	F	Face	2.5	Scalp
581	64	F	Face	1.9	R cheek
582	53	M	Face	1.6	R ear
583	70	F	L limb	3.2	L calf

Table 8.2 (continued)

No	Age	Sex	Region	Diameter (cm)	Location
584	32	F	Trunk	0.3	R breast
585	47	F	Face	0.3	Lower eyelid
586	78	f	Trunk	0.7	R shoulder
587	78	F	Trunk	0.8	L scapular
588	86	F	Face	2	R neck
589	86	F	Face	1.5	Scalp
590	89	F	L limb	2.5	R calf
591	61	M	U limb	1	L ring finger
592	71	F	Face	0.5	Lower eyelid
593	81	F	U limb	1	R ring finger
594	81	f	L limb	2.2	Pre-tibial
595	82	F	U limb	3.6	R forearm
596	54	F	Trunk	0.3	R scapular
597	82	F	Face	2	R scalp
598	82	F	Face	1.8	L scalp
599	82	F	Face	1	Vertex of scalp
600	57	M	L limb	1.5	Pre-tibial
601	57	M	Face	0.1	Lower eyelid
602	74	M	U limb	3.7	R shoulder
603	84	M	Trunk	1.3	Abdominal wall
604	56	M	Face	3	R neck
605	68	M	Face	1.2	Forehead
606	68	M	Face	2.8	Neck
607	86	F	Face	1.8	Left cheek
608	79	M	Face	1	R cheek
609	69	M	Face	2.2	Left temple
610	69	M	Trunk	1.9	Chest
611	49	M	Trunk	0.7	R back
612	64	F	Trunk	0.6	Posterior shoulder
613	64	F	Trunk	1.2	Anterior shoulder
614	67	F	Trunk	2	Back
615	54	M	Trunk	1.2	Lower back
616	74	F	Face	3	Scalp
617	40	F	U limb	2	L forearm
618	54	M	Trunk	1.1	Chest
619	71	F	Trunk	1.7	Back
620	81	M	Face	1.8	Left nose
621	80	M	Face	0.5	Left nose
622	78	M	Face	1.7	Scalp
623	78	M	Trunk	1.7	Left back

(continued)

Table 8.2 (continued)

No	Age	Sex	Region	Diameter (cm)	Location
624	82	M	Face	1.5	Left cheek
625	82	M	face	1.5	Left cheek lower
626	65	F	Face	0.2	Lower eyelid
627	65	F	Face	0.1	Lower eyelid
628	72	F	L limb	1.6	R calf
629	77	F	L limb	1.4	R calf
630	77	F	L limb	1.4	L calf
631	64	M	Trunk	1.7	R scapular
632	72	M	Face	0.6	L cheek
633	57	M	Face	1.1	R lower eyelid
634	95	F	Face	2.3	L cheek
635	49	M	Trunk	2.6	R back
636	62	F	Trunk	0.8	Left breast
637	64	M	Face	1.3	R nose
638	54	M	L limb	6	Right thigh
639	53	M	Face	0.9	Right inner canthus
640	51	M	Face	1.5	Left eyelid
641	37	M	Face	2	R temple
642	74	F	Trunk	1.6	R chest
643	65	F	Face	3.8	L ear
644	57	F	Face	0.4	L anterior nose
645	78	F	Trunk	2.7	L scapular
646	47	F	Face	0.6	Cheek
647	47	F	Trunk	0.8	Chest
648	79	M	Face	5	Scalp
649	60	M	Trunk	1.6	Chest
650	69	M	Face	0.4	R cheek
561	60	F	Lip	0.5	Lower lip
652	72	M	Face	2.5	Scalp
653	51	F	U limb	0.7	L arm
654	25	M	Face	3.5	L neck
655	64	F	Face	1	L cheek
656	77	M	Face	1.2	R neck
657	34	M	Face	2	L temple
658	31	M	U limb	2	R forearm
659	31	M	Trunk	1	Chest
660	31	M	Trunk	1.5	Left chest
661	31	M	Trunk	2	R flank
662	67	M	Trunk	3.2	Scapular
663	55	M	Trunk	0.8	L trapezius
664	72	M	U limb	1.6	R back

Table 8.2 (continued)

No	Age	Sex	Region	Diameter (cm)	Location
665	37	M	Trunk	0.6	R back
666	78	M	Face	2	R ear (graft)
667	49	F	Trunk	0.7	R shoulder
668	70	M	L limb	3.8	L leg
669	70	M	L limb	1.6	L thigh
670	70	M	Trunk	1.6	Scapular
671	70	M	Trunk	2.6	L scapular upper
672	29	F	Trunk	1.2	Abdominal wall
673	51	M	Face	0.3	Right lower eyelid
674	69	F	L limb	2.2	L leg
675	75	M	L limb	2.7	R leg
676	75	M	L limb	2.2	L leg pre-tibial
677	75	M	L limb	1.5	R calf
678	75	M	L limb	1	L knee
679	69	F	L limb	3	R leg
680	57	F	Trunk	1	Upper back
681	50	F	L limb	3.8	L leg
682	78	M	Trunk	1.4	Back
683	45	F	L limb	0.4	L thigh
684	81	M	Trunk	1.8	L chest
685	46	F	L limb	0.4	Pre-tibial
686	78	M	Trunk	2.5	L scapular upper
687	78	M	Trunk	1.2	L scapular lower
688	81	F	L limb	2.7	R leg
689	27	F	Face	1	R neck
690	74	M	Face	0.8	R ear
691	94	M	Trunk	2.8	L back
692	94	M	L limb	2.7	R calf
693	41	F	Face	0.7	R ear
694	73	F	U limb	0.8	L index finger
695	76	M	Face	1	Nose
696	77	F	Face	2.7	Scalp
697	74	M	L limb	2	R thigh
698	47	F	U limb	0.4	Shoulder
699	76	M	Ear	3.8	L ear
700	64	M	U limb	1.4	R arm
701	72	M	Trunk	1.8	R chest
702	77	M	U limb	2.2	R shoulder
703	65	M	Trunk	0.4	L chest
704	83	F	Trunk	2.7	Chest wall
705	62	M	Face	1.8	R neck

(continued)

Table 8.2 (continued)

No	Age	Sex	Region	Diameter (cm)	Location
706	66	M	Trunk	1.6	Back midline
707	66	M	Trunk	2	L scapular
708	61	F	Trunk	0.7	Mid back
709	61	F	Trunk	0.4	Mid back
710	58	F	Trunk	3	L trapezius
711	74	F	U limb	2.2	Left wrist
712	46	F	L limb	2.7	L thigh
713	60	F	U limb	2.2	L index finger
714	62	M	Face	2	Posterior neck
715	81	M	Face	2.2	Forehead
716	61	F	Face	0.3	Nose (biopsy)
717	35	F	L limb	0.6	R little toe
718	65	M	Trunk	1	Upper back
719	62	M	Face	1.2	R neck
720	57	F	L limb	1.6	L leg
721	80	F	L limb	3	L leg
722	69	F	Face	1.8	R cheek
723	69	F	U limb	2	Upper arm
724	63	M	Face	3	R temple
725	68	F	U limb	1.2	R hand
726	75	M	Trunk	4	R back
727	56	F	Face	0.4	Lower eyelid
728	41	F	Face	0.6	R cheek
729	53	F	Face	0.3	Chin
730	60	F	Face	0.3	Upper lip
731	60	M	Trunk	0.5	Upper back
732	52	M	Face	3	Forehead
733	52	M	Face	2.2	R temple
734	52	M	Trunk	2.2	Back
735	55	M	Trunk	0.6	Lower back
736	65	F	Trunk	0.6	Upper back
737	44	F	Trunk	4	R trapezius
738	69	F	Trunk	0.8	R chest
739	78	M	Trunk	2	L abdominal wall
740	56	M	Face	1.5	R neck
741	54	M	Trunk	1.5	Abdominal wall
742	76	F	Trunk	2	Scapular
743	77	F	U limb	2	Left thumb
744	67	F	Face	1.8	Posterior neck
745	54	F	Face	0.5	Neck
746	53	M	Face	0.9	Mucosal lip

Table 8.2   (continued)

No	Age	Sex	Region	Diameter (cm)	Location
747	90	F	Face	2	Scalp
748	74	M	U limb	1.9	R forearm
749	84	F	Face	5	Scalp
750	59	F	Trunk	0.4	R breast
751	58	M	Trunk	1.8	Chest
752	58	M	U limb	1.8	R forearm
753	82	F	Face	4.2	Scalp
754	56	M	U limb	2	L forearm
755	46	F	Face	0.2	Nose
756	65	F	Face	0.7	Lower eyelid
757	57	F	Face	0.5	Nose
758	86	M	Face	1	L lower eyelid
759	50	F	Trunk	1.9	Clavicular
760	63	M	Face	3	Scalp
761	78	M	Trunk	3.2	Chest
762	87	F	U limb	2	Forearm
763	67	F	L limb	1.4	Toenail
764	52	F	Face	0.4	Nose
765	71	M	U limb	1.8	Shoulder
766	81	M	Trunk	2.6	Chest
767	50	m	Scalp	0.5	Scalp
768	50	m	Face	0.5	Ear
769	59	f	Face	2.5	Scalp
770	73	M	Face	2	Ear
771	28	F	U limb	0.5	Forearm
772	28	F	Face	1.5	Forehead
773	83	F	Face	1.6	Nose
774	60	M	Trunk	0.7	Back
775	60	M	Trunk	0.6	Back
776	66	M	Face	1.6	Temple
777	49	M	U limb	1.7	R arm
778	66	F	Trunk	1.5	Upper back
779	68	M	Face	3.2	Forehead
780	70	M	Face	1.7	L cheek
781	27	M	Trunk	0.8	Buttock
782	80	F	Face	1.7	Pre-auricular
783	52	F	Trunk	2	R back
784	52	F	L limb	2.2	R foot
785	71	M	Face	2	L cheek
786	71	M	Face	1.5	Forehead
787	53	F	Face	1	Nose
788	53	F	L limb	1	L leg

(continued)

Table 8.2 (continued)

No	Age	Sex	Region	Diameter (cm)	Location
789	44	F	Face	1.4	Nose
790	69	F	U limb	1.4	R forearm
791	86	M	Face	3	L temple
792	83	f	U limb	3.3	R wrist
793	77	F	U limb	1.4	L hand
794	61	M	Face	1.1	Eyelid
795	73	F	Face	0.8	Eyelid margin
796	73	F	Face	0.3	Lower lip
797	72	M	U limb	0.3	L forearm
798	72	M	L limb	1.2	R leg
799	69	F	Face	1.2	L temple
800	41	F	Trunk	2.3	L trapezius
801	67	F	Face	1.7	Nose
802	49	F	Trunk	0.7	L breast
803	57	M	Face	2.8	L neck
804	57	M	Trunk	2.2	L back
805	64	F	U limb	2	R arm
806	79	M	Trunk	3	Back
807	79	M	L limb	1.6	R leg
808	64	M	Face	0.9	L cheek
809	62	M	Face	1	Forehead
810	43	M	Trunk	0.6	Lower back
811	52	F	Trunk	0.5	Lower back
812	58	M	Face	1	Left neck
813	68	F	L limb	0.5	R thigh
814	66	F	U limb	2	L thigh
815	69	M	Face	2	Left cheek
816	47	F	Trunk	0.7	L groin
817	62	F	U limb	1.7	L forearm
818	63	F	U limb	1.1	L forearm
819	54	F	L limb	1.1	L thigh
820	57	M	Face	1.5	Lower eyelid
821	55	F	Trunk	0.6	Lower back
822	24	F	Trunk	1.5	L breast
823	42	M	Trunk	1.2	Sternum
824	32	F	Face	0.8	Scalp
825	54	F	U limb	2.5	R hand
826	54	F	U limb	1.6	L hand
827	42	f	Face	0.6	L ear
828	51	F	Face	1	Upper lip
829	76	F	Trunk	4	R scapular
830	80	M	L limb	0.9	L leg

Table 8.2 (continued)

No	Age	Sex	Region	Diameter (cm)	Location
831	54	M	Trunk	1.2	R clavicular
832	69	M	Ear	1.8	L ear
833	62	M	Trunk	1.8	R shoulder
834	56	F	Face	1.5	L cheek
835	83	M	Trunk	4.2	L back
836	83	M	Trunk	3.5	R back
837	83	M	Trunk	2.8	Mid back
838	76	M	Face	2.2	L cheek
839	48	F	L Limb	1.8	L thigh
840	46	F	Face	0.5	Forehead
841	46	F	L limb	1.2	R lower leg
842	56	M	Face	1.4	R neck
843	73	M	L Limb	2.2	L temple
844	53	F	Lip	0.2	Lower lip
845	53	F	Trunk	0.3	Upper back
846	76	F	U limb	0.4	Index finger
847	67	M	L limb	2	L ankle
848	44	F	Face	2.2	L nose
849	67	M	Trunk	1.2	R lower back
850	59	M	U limb	1.2	R shoulder
851	62	F	Face	2	R cheek
852	67	F	U limb	1.7	L hand
853	43	M	Trunk	0.5	Abdominal wall
854	25	M	L limb	0.5	R leg
855	48	F	Face	0.5	R neck
856	37	F	Face	0.4	L chin
857	80	M	L limb	1.8	L foot
858	60	F	Trunk	3	L scapular
859	45	F	Face	1	R ala nasi
860	53	F	L limb	3	L leg
861	74	M	Trunk	1.5	R back
862	56	F	Trunk	1	Chest wall
863	85	F	Trunk	1.8	Chest wall
864	59	F	Face	0.5	R cheek
865	63	F	Trunk	0.6	Back
866	52	M	Trunk	3	L back
867	39	M	Face	0.3	Scalp
868	77	M	Face	1.8	L temple
869	57	F	Lip	0.3	Lower lip
870	56	M	Trunk	0.5	Chest
871	70	F	Trunk	1.3	Back
872	69	M	Face	1.2	R forehead

(continued)

Table 8.2 (continued)

No	Age	Sex	Region	Diameter (cm)	Location
873	68	F	Face	3	L neck
874	88	M	Trunk	2.2	L scapular
875	32	F	L limb	0.8	L big toe
876	53	M	Trunk	0.7	Scapular
877	81	M	U limb	1.1	R elbow
878	83	M	Face	1.3	R ear
879	83	M	Face	1.4	R cheek
880	32	F	Face	0.2	Lower lip
881	61	F	U limb	0.9	L upper arm
882	15	M	Trunk	0.6	L chest
883	66	F	L limb	0.7	R knee
884	72	M	Face	0.3	R eyelid
885	75	M	Trunk	2.5	R scapular
886	75	M	Face	0.8	R cheek
887	28	F	Face	0.3	Cheek
888	28	F	Trunk	0.4	Chest
889	30	F	Face	0.5	L ear
890	71	F	Face	1.4	Nose
891	45	F	Face	1.7	R cheek
892	67	M	Trunk	1.4	L scapular
893	64	F	Trunk	1	Chest
894	64	F	Trunk	1.6	Upper back
895	64	F	Trunk	2	Mid back
896	42	F	L limb	1.1	L upper thigh
897	62	M	Face	1.2	L cheek
898	70	M	Trunk	1.2	L chest
899	70	M	Trunk	1	L scapular
900	80	M	U limb	1.5	R arm lower
901	80	M	U limb	1	R arm upper
902	82	M	U limb	1.2	L forearm
903	82	M	U limb	2.7	R arm
904	72	M	Face	1.2	Nose
905	76	M	U limb	1.8	R hand
906	76	M	U limb	2.1	R shoulder
907	30	F	Face	0.5	Upper lip
908	55	M	Face	2.2	L cheek
909	56	M	Face	0.5	L neck
910	69	M	Face	1.1	R scalp
911	23	F	Lip	0.5	Lower lip
912	68	M	Face	0.4	L ear
913	52	F	Face	1.2	R nose
914	59	F	Trunk	1.6	Upper back

Table 8.2   (continued)

No	Age	Sex	Region	Diameter (cm)	Location
915	73	M	Face	4	L cheek
916	57	M	Face	4	L neck
917	82	F	U limb	1.2	L thumb
918	76	M	Trunk	3	Chest
919	78	F	L limb	2	L thigh
920	71	M	U limb	2.2	R forearm
921	66	F	U limb	0.4	L elbow
922	66	F	Trunk	0.7	R scapular
923	74	M	Trunk	4.6	Back
924	64	F	Trunk	1.2	Chest
925	87	F	Face	1.2	Cheek
926	48	F	Trunk	4	Back
927	48	F	Face	0.4	Lower eyelid
928	63	F	Trunk	1.5	Chest
929	56	M	Face	2.8	R neck
930	50	M	U limb	2	Forearm
931	50	M	U limb	1.3	L arm
932	81	F	U limb	1.6	L forearm
933	78	F	L limb	0.6	L calf
934	69	M	Face	1.2	L flank
935	70	F	Face	0.2	Nose
936	76	M	Face	2.2	L cheek
937	22	F	Trunk	0.3	Pubic region
938	81	F	Trunk	2	Scapular
939	81	F	Trunk	1.5	R shoulder
940	28	M	Trunk	2.9	Mid back
941	79	M	Trunk	2	R back
942	28	M	Face	1.2	Scalp
943	75	M	Trunk	0.6	Mid back
944	56	M	Face	2	Neck
945			U limb	2.5	R arm
946	75	M	U limb	2	R forearm
947	41	F	Face	0.3	L cheek
948	78	M	U limb	1.2	L hand
949	68	F	Face	3	L neck
950	88	M	Trunk	2.2	Scapular
951	30	F	Face	0.2	Lip
952	67	M	Trunk	4	Back
953	52	F	Trunk	2.5	Chest
954	69	F	Face	2.8	Neck
955	76	F	U limb	2.7	R hand
956	72	F	L limb	1.4	L leg

(continued)

Table 8.2 (continued)

No	Age	Sex	Region	Diameter (cm)	Location
957			U limb	1	R hand
958	72	F	Face	1.8	Cheek
959	52	M	Trunk	2.4	Back
960	44	F	Trunk	3.4	L scapular
961	68	F	Face	3.2	Cheek
962			Trunk	1.2	Upper back
963	70	M	Face	0.5	Lower eyelid
964	80	M	Trunk	0.4	R scapular
965			L Limb	3.5	Calf
966	75	M	Trunk	0.3	Upper back
967	79	M	Trunk	1.3	L back
968	87	M	U limb	3.7	R forearm
969	55	F	Trunk	1.9	Sternum
970	55	F	Face	1.8	Anterior scalp
971			Face	2	Posterior scalp
972	80	M	Trunk	5	L chest
973			Trunk	1.9	R back
974	85	F	Face	1	Neck
975	69	M	Trunk	2.2	R chest
976			Trunk	2	L scapular
977	25	M	L limb	2.2	R leg
978	55	F	U limb	1.8	R hand
979	46	M	Face	0.5	R nose
980	56	F	Face	1	R cheek
981	56	F	Face	0.4	Lower lip
982	72	M	Trunk	1.6	Upper back
983	51	F	Face	1.3	L cheek
984	71	M	Trunk	1.4	Mid back
985	43	M	Trunk	1.5	R scapular
986	43	M	Face	2.5	R cheek
987	74	F	trunk	1.8	R back
988	68	F	U limb	2	L arm
989	73	M	Face	0.8	R ear
990	73	M	Face	1.1	L ear
991	76	M	L limb	1.8	L knee
992	78	M	L limb	5	L calf
993	78	M	Trunk	3.5	Chest
994	75	F	U limb	1.8	L forearm
995	75	M	L limb	1.7	L leg
996	74	M	Trunk	1	Chest
997			Face	0.9	Ear
998	75	F	L limb	0.7	L leg

Table 8.2 (continued)

No	Age	Sex	Region	Diameter (cm)	Location
999	62	F	U limb	2.2	Forearm
1000	87	M	L limb	2.7	L leg
1001	55	M	Face	1.2	Neck
1002	51	M	L limb	0.5	R big toe
1003	59	M	Face	0.7	L cheek
1004	39	M	Trunk	0.4	Lower back
1005	74	M	Trunk	1.8	L back
1006	39	M	Trunk	4	R buttock
1007	70	M	Trunk	1.5	Chest
1008	33	M	Face	0.3	Temple
1009	61	F	L limb	1.5	R calf
1010	74	M	Trunk	3.3	Mid back
1011	70	M	Ear	1.8	L ear
1012	49	F	Face	3.2	Nose
1013	65	M	Trunk	4	Back
1014	67	F	Face	2	L cheek
1015	68	M	Face	1	Forehead
1016	63	M	Face	1.7	Scalp
1017	63	M	Trunk	0.7	Back
1018	67	F	Trunk	1	Scapula
1019	45	F	L limb	0.7	R calf
1020	45	F	L limb	0.4	R leg
1021	43	F	Lip	0.2	Lower lip
1022	59	F	Trunk	0.5	Mid back
1023	59	F	Trunk	1	L back
1024	84	M	Face	2.5	Ear
1025	86	F	Face	1.9	Lower eyelid
1026	41	F	Trunk	0.7	R back
1027	47	F	L limb	1.2	R thigh
1028	83	F	L limb	2.7	L leg
1029	56	F	U limb	0.2	Index finger
1030	56	F	U limb	0.4	Axilla
1031	57	M	Face	0.9	L temple
1032	52	f	Trunk	3	R buttock
1033	76	M	L limb	2.4	L leg
1034	63	F	Face	1	R cheek
1035	63	M	Trunk	2.4	Abdominal wall
1036	82	F	Trunk	1.4	Left back
1037	82	F	Trunk	1.9	Left back
1038	59	F	Face	0.4	Cheek
1039	41	F	Face	0.7	R neck
1040	41	F	Face	0.6	L neck

(continued)

Table 8.2 (continued)

No	Age	Sex	Region	Diameter (cm)	Location
1041	41	F	U limb	0.3	R hand
1042	83	F	U Limb	2.8	L arm
1043	71	M	Trunk	0.7	Scapular
1044	71	M	Trunk	0.4	Trunk
1045	72	M	Face	1	Cheek
1046	73	F	Face	0.4	Cheek
1047	73	F	Face	0.5	Chin
1048	77	M	Face	2	Forehead
1049	61	M	Face	3.3	Neck
1050	80	F	Face	0.8	Cheek
1051	38	F	Trunk	1.1	Chest wall
1052	72	M	U limb	2	R forearm
1053	75	F	Trunk	1.8	R breast
1054	68	M	Trunk	0.7	R flank
1055	59	F	Trunk	1.5	Upper back
1056	59	F	Trunk	0.9	Mid back
1057	88	F	L limb	1.7	R ankle
1058	35	M	L limb	1	R thigh
1059	60	F	Trunk	1	Trapezius
1060	58	F	Face	1.7	Forehead
1061	45	M	Face	1.8	Temple
1062	80	F	Face	2.8	Ear
1063	67	F	Trunk	1	Back
1064	83	F	Trunk	0.6	Upper back
1065	22	F	Scalp	1	Scalp
1066	64	F	Face	0.5	L neck
1067	64	F	Face	0.6	R neck
1068	88	F	L limb	3	R ankle
1069	80	F	Face	0.7	Forehead
1070	80	F	Face	0.7	L cheek
1071	65	M	Face	1	Neck
1072	65	M	Face	1.5	L forearm
1073	75	F	Face	0.8	R ear
1074	61	M	Face	2	Lower eyelid
1075	47	F	Face	0.4	Cheek
1076	54	M	L limb	2.5	R thigh
1077	77	F	U limb	1.1	Forearm
1078	59	M	Face	2.5	Forehead
1079	89	M	Trunk	0.7	Back
1080	74	M	L limb	3.5	Lower leg
1081	84	M	Face	2.8	R temple
1082	46	F	Trunk	0.4	Trunk

Table 8.2 (continued)

No	Age	Sex	Region	Diameter (cm)	Location
1083	40	M	Trunk	0.8	L shoulder
1084	40	M	U limb	0.5	R chest
1085	54	F	L limb	0.4	Popliteal fossa
1086	39	F	Lip	0.4	Lower lip
1087	72	F	L limb	1.8	L thigh
1088	75	M	Face	2	Scalp
1089	75	M	Face	2.5	Forehead
1090	75	M	Face	2.2	Scalp
1091	75	M	Trunk	1.8	Chest
1092	74	F	Ear	0.7	Ear
1093	74	F	Face	0.5	Nose
1094	61	M	Trunk	2.5	Chest
1095	40	M	Trunk	1	Abdominal wall
1096	59	F	L limb	0.4	L foot
1097	69	M	Trunk	2.2	Upper back
1098	48	F	Trunk	1.7	Chest
1099	47	F	Trunk	3	Neck
1100	64	M	Ear	2.5	Ear
1101	64	M	Trunk	1.2	Trunk
1102	65	M	Ear	2	Tragus
1103	65	M	Face	2	Scalp
1104	77	F	L limb	6	L calf
1105	74	M	Face	0.7	Eye
1106	74	M	Ear	0.8	Ear
1107	72	M	Face	2.5	Cheek
1108	62	M	Trunk	1.2	Shoulder
1109	58	M	Face	1.2	Lower eyelid
1110	72	F	U limb	2.2	Posterior arm
1111	68	M	U limb	2	Arm
1112	66	M	Trunk	0.6	Mid back
1113	42	F	Trunk	0.9	Upper back
1114	52	F	Trunk	2.2	Thigh
1115	76	M	Trunk	2.5	R back
1116	81	M	Trunk	1.6	Upper back
1117	81	M	Trunk	2	Lower back
1118	66	F	Face	0.4	Lower eyelid
1119	86	F	L limb	3	Pre-tibial R leg
1120	80	M	Trunk	2.5	Back
1121	69	F	Trunk	1.7	Chest
1122	62	M	Scalp	3.2	Scalp
1123	71	F	Trunk	0.8	Sacral
1124	71	F	Face	0.4	Temple

(continued)

Table 8.2 (continued)

No	Age	Sex	Region	Diameter (cm)	Location
1125	80	F	Face	1.2	R cheek
1126	90	F	L limb	1.3	R calf
1127	24	M	Trunk	0.4	Abdominal wall
1128	74	F	Face	2	Nose
1129	71	M	L limb	3.2	L leg
1130	54	M	Face	0.9	Eyelid
1131	70	M	Face	1.6	Cheek
1132	51	F	Face	0.4	Scalp
1133	58	F	Trunk	1.4	Upper back
1134	42	F	Trunk	0.7	Upper back
1135	64	M	Trunk	1.8	Upper back
1136	64	M	Trunk	1.8	R scapular
1137	78	M	Trunk	2	L scapular
1138	78	M	Face	2.2	Ear
1139	74	M	Face	2.5	Scalp
1140	74	M	L limb	2.5	R thigh
1141	67	M	Face	1	L lower eyelid
1142	58	F	Face	1	L cheek
1143	28	M	Face	0.8	R cheek
1144	28	M	Face	0.4	L cheek
1145	63	F	Face	0.4	R nose
1146	63	F	L limb	0.3	L lower leg
1147	66	M	Trunk	2	Chest
1148	38	F	Face	0.4	Cheek
1149	84	M	Face	1.8	L cheek
1150	50	F	Face	1.8	L cheek
1151	62	M	L limb	4.6	L calf
1152	47	M	Trunk	2	L trapezius
1153	44	F	Trunk	1	L clavicular
1154	39	F	U limb	0.5	R upper arm
1155	62	M	Face	1.5	R cheek
1156	39	M	Face	0.5	R cheek
1157	74	M	Trunk	2.3	R chest
1157	74	M	Trunk	1.2	L chest
1157	78	M	Face	1.4	R lower eyelid
1158	56	F	Face	0.6	Forehead
1159	62	M	L limb	1.9	R thigh
1160	44	M	Trunk	0.7	Midline upper back
1161	62	M	Trunk	2.4	R back
1162	69	M	Face	3.2	L neck
1163	75	M	Face	2.5	Forehead

Table 8.2 (continued)

No	Age	Sex	Region	Diameter (cm)	Location
1164	67	M	Face	5	R neck
1165	75	F	Face	1.6	Lower lip
1166	77	F	Face	2.2	Scalp
1167	80	M	Face	1.2	R temple
1168	80	M	Trunk	1.2	L scapular
1169	44	F	Face	1	Posterior neck
1170	66	M	Face	1.7	Forehead
1171	74	M	L limb	0.7	R thigh
1172	47	F	Face	1	Scalp
1173	42	F	Face	0.4	Cheek
1174	76	M	Face	3.5	R forehead
1175	76	M	Trunk	1.2	Back
1176	65	F	Ear	1.6	Infra-auricular
1177	20	F	Trunk	0.5	R buttock
1178	38	M	U limb	7	Posterior Shoulder
1179	32	M	Trunk	4	R flank
1180	64	M	Trunk	3.4	Upper back
1181	69	F	U limb	2.5	L forearm
	64.12048878 (mean age)			1.624619289 (average size in cm)	

shrinkage and ranged from 0.4 to 4.5 cm with an average size of 1.62 cm. It has already been reported that for defects under 0.8 cm, there seems to be no preferential direction with respect to reduced wound tension [19]. BEST line wound tension measurements have been published previously [18, 19]. Therefore, in this chapter, individual wound tension measurements are not the focus, as is the mapping of the direction of closure under least tension (BEST line). Given the large number of lesions, the idea was to present a map of BEST lines across the body as a guide for surgical excisions of skin cancer or skin lesions.

Once lesions were excised in a circular fashion and best line of closure determined, the wounds were converted into an elliptical excision on the trunk and limbs based on BEST lines (Fig. 8.1). The direction of ellipse to allow for closure under least tension (BEST line) was mapped. All excisions were full thickness skin specimens and removal of neoplastic lesions usually involved excision of some underlying fat. All lesions were sent for histopathological examination wherein the measurements of the samples were taken (in the Table 8.2) after tissue shrinkage in formalin.

The degree of tissue shrinkage after surgery has been a subject of conjecture with many different authors looking at this issue. Dauendorffer and colleagues reported that the shrinkage of skin excision specimens occurred immediately after surgical excision and prior to formalin fixation [20]. They reported that mean *in vivo* and *in vitro* shrinkages were 16% for length and 18% for width ($p < 0.001$); while tissue shrinkage occurred in both *in vivo* and *ex vivo* measurements ($p < 0.001$), there was no difference noted between these measurements. Importantly, the authors concluded that after adjusting for initial width, width shrinkage was neither significantly associated with the type of lesion (malignant or not, $p = 0.20$), nor with the location on the trunk ($p = 0.35$) [20]. Other studies by Kerns looking at tissue shrinkage suggest that patient age is significant, and tissue shrinkage decreases 0.3% per year of increasing age, but the body site of the specimen was not significant [21]. These studies suggest that cutaneous tissue shrinkage following excision is primarily because of intrinsic tissue contractility, and solar elastosis due to age also correlates with less shrinkage [21]. In our study, the mean diameter of excision specimen was 1.62 cm (and maximum diameter 4.5 cm) *after* tissue shrinkage and formalin fixation.

The site of each lesion and the direction of closure along BEST lines was mapped and the images (Figs. 8.2 and 8.3) give a good idea of biodynamic excisional skin tension (BEST) lines across the body i.e. the lines to be followed to achieve closure under least tension (Fig. 8.4). All procedures were performed by one surgeon (the author) and this study was of 1181 consecutive (excisional) lesions. We had aimed for 1500 lesions but our tensiometer suffered a malfunction at the 1181 lesion mark and therefore the study was stopped at this point to ensure accuracy. This was the last tensiometer prototype developed for this PhD study project and building a new device was not feasible due to time and cost constraints, especially as this study plan involved consecutive lesions that needed excisional surgery. However, this still represents the largest series reported in any skin-line study and the only *in vivo* real-time surgical study (Table 8.1).

Karl Langer, who originally investigated cleavage lines studied cadavers that were punctured with an awl, a device not dissimilar to an ice-pick [22]. Langer published a series of papers in 1861 that were not translated until 1978 by Gibson [22]. Cox, who recreated Langer's experiment in 1941, studied 28 cadavers on which numerous puncture wounds had been created [23]. Because Borges's proposed pinch method [24] to elucidate RSTL is not accurate on the trunk, many skin tension studies have been undertaken—however these studies have all involved a very small number of cadavers or animals. For example, a recent study of two dogs used a Reviscometer to study elastic waves of skin to understand skin tension lines [25]. Given the small size of all previous studies, and the lack of actual real-time measurements during surgery, the author is pleased to present for the first time a large consecutive *in vivo* real-time surgical series as part of this inquisition into the BEST lines for surgical excisions.

In general, on the trunk, BEST lines run in a horizontal direction; on the limbs they run vertically—and overall they show a remarkable consistency of pattern as seen in the images. On the shoulder and scapular regions, especially laterally, there appears to be a more vertical orientation, and the fibres appear more oblique (Fig. 8.4). This is in keeping with the findings of several experiments [26, 27] using well known *in vitro* test methods such as the Kolsky bar, also known as a split Hopkinson pressure bar. Such studies [26, 27] on pigskin samples have shown that

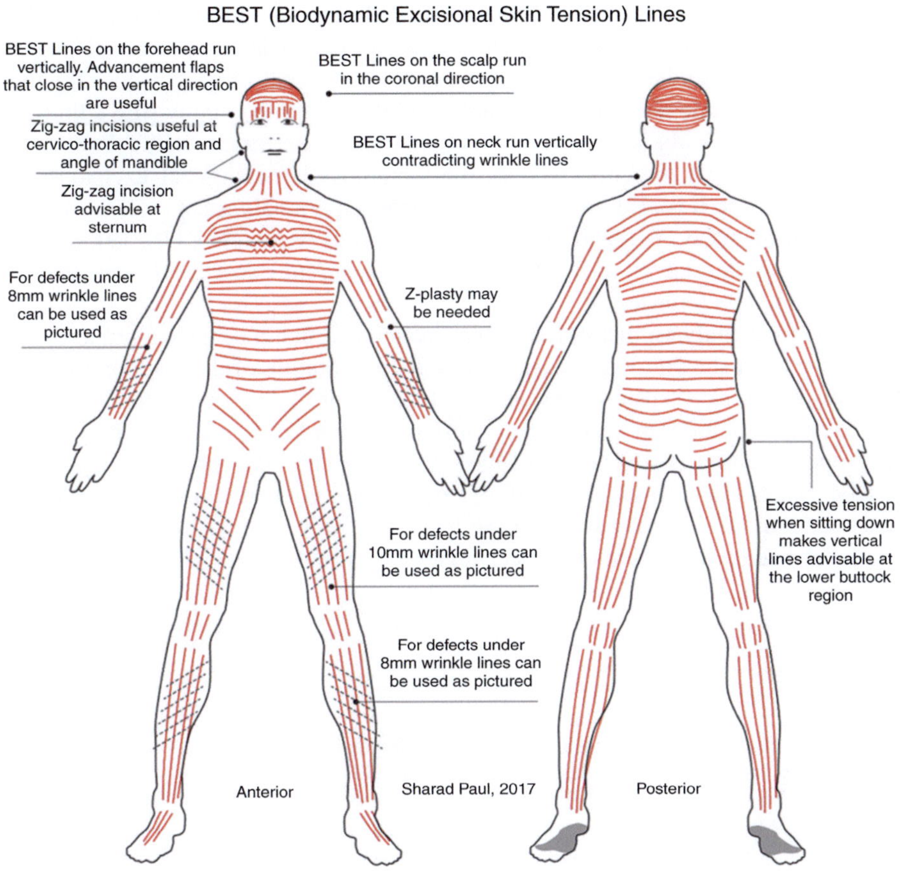

Fig. 8.4 BEST lines to guide surgical excisions

pigskin exhibits rate-sensitive, non-linear behaviour whose properties can vary with respect to spinal orientation—while other studies have already confirmed that the superficial fascial system of pigskin and human skin behave the same mechanically [16].

In studying the mechanism of wrinkle line formation, authors have noted that spontaneous contraction of the dermis while maintaining or increasing the epidermal area induces buckling of the epidermis into the dermis at mechanically weak lines, namely, the rows of pores and sulci cutis, and this is amplified by the axial compression of the dermis by the muscle layer [28]. However, as discussed in other chapters, wrinkle lines have no advantage in handling skin stress and that is why BEST lines matter most of all [29].

The biomechanics of limbs, especially the upper limb have been extensively studied. Under conditions of low physical stress, there is a thinning of forearm skin parallel to the forearm axis and thickening of forearm skin perpendicular to the forearm axis; however, under conditions seen in excisional surgery i.e. higher-stress, these findings are reversed [30]. This is not unlike this author's findings regarding the interplay between collagen and elastin during incisional and excisional surgery [31]. What these studies also reiterate is that for excisional surgery, especially after skin cancer, wrinkle lines are not suitable, and it is better to employ BEST lines.

In distal (below the knee and elbow) upper and lower limbs, BEST lines again run in the vertical direction and are best employed for surgical excisions. As described earlier, it is also important to close the superficial fascial system and nullify any dead space. As noted by the author in previous chapters [18, 19], under a 7–8 mm diameter defect, or for defects not involving the complete dermis, there is no directional preference.

In the final analysis, many studies have concluded that mechanical properties of skin have been shown to vary according to the orientation of the loading direction with respect to skin tension lines, and the location of the lesions or the position of the subject's shoulder or scapula can cause confusion [32]. To achieve best results post-operatively, it is advisable to follow BEST lines, and to close the superficial fascial system—and this chapter offers a directional guide to close a wound under least tension and reduce scar width. Some of this research into BEST lines of the trunk has been presented in other peer-reviewed journal articles [33].

References

1. Paul SP, et al. A new skin tensiometer device: computational analyses to understand biodynamic excisional skin tension lines. Sci Rep. 2016;6:30117.
2. Bush J, Ferguson MWJ, et al. The dynamic rotation of Langer's lines on facial expression. JPRAS. 2007;60:393–9.
3. Langer K. On the anatomy and physiology of the skin I. The cleavability of the cutis. Br J Plast Surg. 1978;31:3–8.
4. Simon HK, Zempsky WT, Bruns TB, et al. Lacerations against Langer's lines: to glue or suture? J Emerg Med. 1998;16(2):185–9.
5. Son D, Harijan A. Overview of surgical scar prevention and management. J Korean Med Sci. 2014;29(6):751–7.
6. Bayat A, McGrouther DA, Ferguson MW. Skin scarring. BMJ. 2003;326:88–92.
7. Monstrey S, Middelkoop E, Vranckx JJ, et al. Updated scar management practical guidelines: non-invasive and invasive measures. JPRAS. 2014;67(8):1017–25.
8. Young VL, Hutchison J. Insights into patient and clinician concerns about scar appearance: semi-quantitative structured surveys. Plast Reconstr Surg. 2009;124:256–65.
9. Kumar N, Kumar P, et al. Quantitative fraction evaluation of dermal collagen and elastic fibres in the skin samples obtained in two orientations from the trunk region. Dermatol Res Pract. 2014;2014:251254.
10. Paul SP. The use of zigs and zags to reduce scarring over "Keloid triangles" during excisional surgery: biomechanics, review and recommendations. Surg Sci. 2017;8:240–55.
11. Lockwood TE. Superficial fascial system (SFS) of the trunk and extremities: a new concept. Plast Reconstr Surg. 1991;87:1009–18.
12. Pollock H, Pollock T. Progressive tension sutures: a technique to reduce local complications in abdominoplasty. Plast Reconstr Surg. 2000;105:2583–6.
13. Topaz M, Carmel N-N, Silberman A, Li MS, Li YZ. The TopClosure® 3S system, for skin stretching and a secure wound closure. Eur J Plast Surg. 2012;35(7):533–43.

14. Saffle JI. The phenomenon of "fluid creep" in acute burn resuscitation. J Burn Care Res. 2007;28(3):382–95.
15. Ismavel R, et al. A simple solution for wound coverage by skin stretching. J Orthop Trauma. 2011;25(3):127–32.
16. Song AY, Askari M, et al. Biomechanical properties of the superficial fascial system. Aesthet Surg J. 2006;4:395–403.
17. Wilhemi BJ, Blackwell SJ, Mancoll JS, Phillips LG. Creep vs stretch: a review of the viscoelastic properties of skin. Ann Plast Surg. 1998;41:215–9.
18. Paul SP. The golden spiral flap: a new flap design that allows for closure of larger wounds under reduced tension—how studying nature's own design led to the development of a new surgical technique. Front Surg. 2016;3:63.
19. Paul SP. Revisiting Langer's lines, introducing best lines, and studying the biomechanics of scalp skin. Spectr Dermatol. 2017;2:8–11.
20. Dauendorffer JN, Bastuji-Garin S, Guéro S, Brousse N, Fraitag S. Shrinkage of skin excision specimens: formalin fixation is not the culprit. Br J Dermatol. 2009;160(4):810–4.
21. Kerns MJ, Darst MA, Olsen TG, Fenster M, Hall P, Grevey S. Shrinkage of cutaneous specimens: formalin or other factors involved? J Cutan Pathol. 2008;35(12):1093–6.
22. Langer K. Zur Anatomie und Physiologie der Haut. I) Ueber die Spaltbarkeit der Cutis; 2) Die Spannung der Cutis; 3) Ueber die Elasticita der Cutis; 4) Das Quellungvermogen der Cutis. Sitzzungsbericht der Mathematisch-natunvissenschaftlichen Classe der Kaiserlichen Academia der Wissenschaften, Wien, 1861. [From: On the anatomy and physiology of the skin. Br J Plast Surg. 31:3–8, 93–106. 185–199, 273–278, 1978.1].
23. Cox HT. The cleavage lines of the skin. Br J Surg. 1941;29:234–40.
24. Borges AF. Relaxed skin tension lines (RSTL) versus other skin lines. Plast Reconstr Surg. 1984;73:144–50.
25. Deroy C, Destrade M, McAlinden A, Ni Annaidh A. Non-invasive evaluation of skin tension lines with elastic waves. Med Phys 2016;1–14. arXiv:1609.07267.
26. Lim J, Hong J, Chen WW, Weerasooriya T. Mechanical response of pig skin under dynamic tensile loading. Int J Impact Eng. 2001;38:130–5.
27. Shergold OA, Fleck NA, Radford D. The uniaxial stress versus strain response of pig skin and silicone rubber at low and high strain rates. Int J Impact Eng. 2004;32:1384–402.
28. Matsumoto T. Biomechanics of wrinkle formation. J Jpn Cosmetic Sci Soc. 2013;37(2):101–6.
29. Paul SP. Biodynamic excisional skin tension (best) lines: revisiting Langer's lines, skin biomechanics, current concepts in cutaneous surgery, and the (lack of) science behind skin lines used for surgical excisions. J Dermatol Res. 2017;2(1):77–87.
30. Gahagnon S, et al. Skin anisotropy in vivo and initial natural stress effect: a quantitative study using high-frequency static elastography. J Biomech. 2012;45:2860–5.
31. Paul SP. Are incisional and excisional skin tension lines biomechanically different? Understanding the interplay between elastin and collagen during surgical procedures. Int J Biomed. 2017;7(2):111–4.
32. Gallagher AJ, Anniadh N, Bruyere K, Otténio M, Xie H, Gilchrist MD. Dynamic tensile properties of human skin. In: IRCOBI conference. 2012; IRC. 12: 59, 494–500.
33. Paul SP. Biodynamic excisional skin tension (BEST) lines for surgical excisions: untangling the science. Ann R Coll Surg Engl. 2018;1–8.

Chapter 9
BEST Lines of the Lower Limb

9.1 Introduction

The lower limb presents an interesting reconstructive challenge because the "surgical plane" of the lower limb lies deep to deep fascia—dye-injection studies done by Haertsch [1] on 22 post-mortem legs demonstrated the role of the fascial plexus. His study showed that the fascial plexus communicated with the sub-dermal plexus, and sometimes with a vascular plexus on the underside of the deep fascia. Excisions after skin cancer are even more significant on the leg—a site known to have higher degrees of wound complications [2, 3]. Further, in 5–10% of skin cancers, adjuvant treatments such as radiotherapy or chemotherapy are needed to counteract neoplastic growth—significantly compromising local tissue vascularization [4]. Many other factors can delay wound healing or cause wound dehiscence in oncological patients, such as a high body mass index, immunosuppressive disorders, diabetes, peripheral vascular disease and tobacco use [5]. Patients that have undergone radiation treatment can have wound complications later, due to radiation inhibiting fibroblasts outgrowth, reducing deposition of collagen and wound strength, and decreasing angiogenesis [4].

A lower leg wound is defined as being chronic if it has failed to heal (i.e. achieved anatomical and functional integrity) within 3 months, and ulcers following wound breakdown are more common on the lower limb [6]. Diabetes mellitus slows wound maturation and decreases numbers of dermal fibroblasts, as does a slightly raised HbA1C [7]. In a study involving plastic surgical procedures such as flaps, it was noted that 1 pack-per-day smokers had three times the frequency of necrosis, and 2 pack-per-day smokers had six times the frequency of necrosis when compared to non-smokers [8]. Angiosomes need to be considered during incision placement [9] and vertically placed incisions in the lower leg have less danger to angiosomes as they can be placed at junctions between angiosomes. Vascularity of the lower limb will be discussed in detail in another chapter in this book. Sutures and suture techniques for skin closure need to be considered in the lower limb

© Springer International Publishing AG, part of Springer Nature 2018
S. P. Paul, *Biodynamic Excisional Skin Tension Lines for Cutaneous Surgery*,
https://doi.org/10.1007/978-3-319-71495-0_9

given the higher wound infection risk. In general, monofilament sutures are preferable for skin closure, and sutures should not be too tight—allowing for the postoperative swelling of tissues to reduce ischaemia risk [10]. It is therefore even more important to understand biodynamic excisional skin tension (BEST) lines on the lower limb—lines of orientation that allow a wound to be closed under the least possible tension.

The goal of lower extremity reconstruction (after skin cancer excision, for example) is the complete removal of tumours and the coverage of resultant defects, to deliver patients a healed wound, and to let them resume work and recreation [11]. When wounds are small, primary closure is feasible; however, when wounds are too large to be closed primarily, in addition to traditional partial and full thickness skin grafts [12], halo grafts [13], perforator island flaps such as the Keystone Design flap [14] and reducing opposed multi-lobed (ROM) flaps [15] have been described previously. For extremely large wounds, free tissue transfer [16] is often employed.

While closure of wounds under least tension is well known to result in best outcomes to do with both wound healing and scar formation, the lines of excision that result in least tension have often been contentious. It has been noted by this author earlier that many textbooks depict skin tension lines such as Langer's Lines differently, and there may be a "lack of science behind skin lines currently used for surgical excisions" [17].

Borges first described the concept of using relaxed skin tension lines (RSTL) for excisions of skin lesions on the face. RSTL are based on the concept that when skin is relaxed, furrows are formed—and these lines are made more noticeable by pinching skin and noting the direction of furrows and ridges [18]. However, on the rest of the body or areas such as the lower limb, Borges generally referred to Kraissl's lines [19] which are essentially wrinkle lines. Recently, after studies on wound tension in surgical wounds, this author proposed the hypothesis that incisional and excisional lines need to be considered differently [20]. Wrinkle lines that may be suitable for surgical incisions are not necessarily load-bearing enough to allow them to handle the increased loads of excisional surgery [21].

From a bioengineering perspective, skin is a composite material that behaves elastically only at low-load levels. In areas like the lower limb and feet, as discussed earlier, due to increased weight-bearing functions, skin is increasingly viscoelastic i.e. strain becomes a function of load and time [21]. In sun-damaged lower limbs, while changes due to age are visible to the observer, the underlying elastin network also shows degradation over time [22].

On the lower limb, especially below the knee, the consequence of improperly oriented initial excision-lines is greater, as it may mean the difference between primary closure or the need for a skin graft—with its associated longer healing time and suboptimal cosmetic result. Therefore, getting the orientation of an ellipse correct while planning excisional surgery is of paramount importance. In this chapter, the author studies the best orientation of ellipses on the lower limb (below knee) for skin lesion excisions—a study that led to the development of a new technique of lowering wound tension using parallel relaxing incisions.

9.2   Materials and Methods

Surgical Procedure: This study was done using a tensiometer to measure tension after defects were cut out in a circular fashion, with no pre-determined direction of closure. Studies using this tensiometer on different body sites have already shown that under a diameter of 7–8 mm, there is very little differences in wound-closing tension [23]. While it has been often discussed that skin is anisotropic, in areas close to the bone like the pretibial region, it does exhibit orthotropy i.e. a degree of symmetry with respect to two normal planes, which is thought to be due to the preferential orientation of collagen fibres [24]. Therefore, this study ended up a test of the hypothesis: Vertically-oriented excisions have less wound-closing tension when compared to oblique or RSTL/wrinkle line wound closures. Twenty-three circular lower limb defects with diameters ranging from 1.5 to 4.5 cm were studied as detailed in the table below.

Tensiometer: The development and design of the tensiometer used for this study (Fig. 9.1) has been described in detail in a previous chapter and paper [20]. The device is made up of four main elements, a linear actuator, a force sensor, signal conditioning hardware and embedded software: The linear actuator provides a

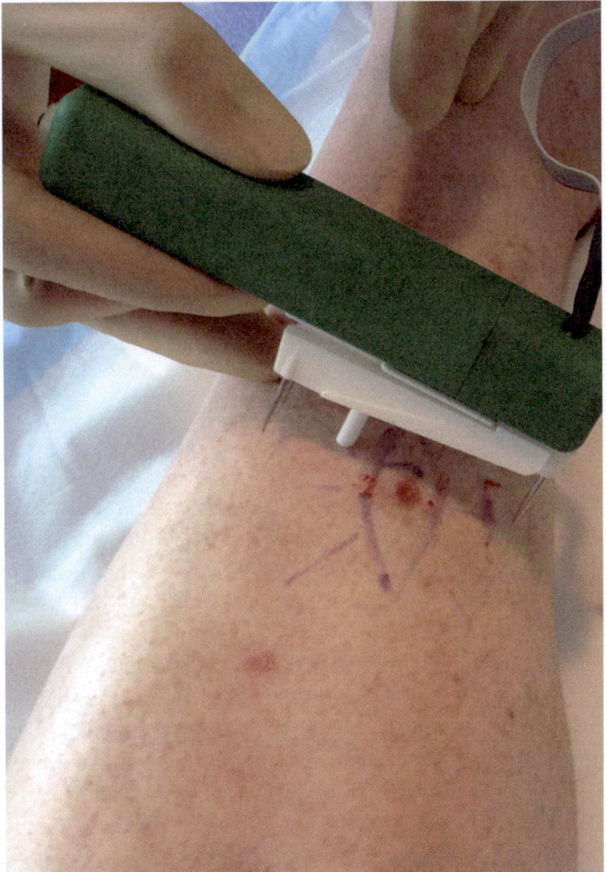

Fig. 9.1 Measuring tension along different directions using a specially designed tensiometer

consistent force that is applied to the skin to measure wound tension, with a special focus on wound closing tension. The force sensor is a strain-element force-sensor and has a sensing range of 0–10 Newton's (N) that has been deemed an adequate range in previous skin tension studies [20]. The force needed to bring the wound edges together after a defect is created is converted to a proportional voltage potential, and passed through signal conditioning software. The embedded software provides control for the linear actuator and converts the signal voltage from the force sensor into measurable tension, that is displayed on the instrument panel. This device was bi-directional, i.e., this allowed the author to measure inward and outward forces by flicking the switch to change the direction of measurement—allowing for the assessment of inherent skin tension (pre-tension), and wound-closing tension [20].

A formal study on patients was undertaken, after obtaining all the necessary ethics approvals [New Zealand Health and Disability Ethics Committee (HDEC Reference number 15/CEN/113); Australia: University of Queensland Institutional Human Ethics (Approval No. 2015001550)]. This study was carried out in accordance with the recommendations of the ethics committees listed above, with written informed consent from all subjects. All subjects gave written informed consent in accordance with the Declaration of Helsinki. All patients presented for skin cancer surgery and were operated upon by a single surgeon (in this case the author). Twenty-one consecutive patients underwent 23 procedures. Two patients had two lesions (and one of them had identical-sized lesions on both pretibial regions allowing for a biomechanical comparison between the parallel fascia-relaxing incision and a Type 1 keystone island perforator flap [4] that was used on the other limb).

Closing wound tension was measured before and after the wounds were excised in a circular fashion, and pre-tension was also measured prior to the excision (Fig. 9.1). The measurements were compared along the RSTL and the vertical plane—because these two directions had the lowest tension measurements consistently, compared to other directions—confirming that in areas like the lower limb, skin exhibits orthotropy rather than anisotropy.

9.3 Results

Twenty-one patients aged between 50 and 88 underwent 23 operations. There were 13 males and 8 female patients. All excisions were for sizeable skin neoplasms and the diameters of the circular defects created are noted in Table 9.1 below.

The tension force measurements are noted in Newtons (N) in the table above. A detailed statistical analysis was undertaken. Nos. 1 and 2 were the same patient, a 69-year old male who had a 3.5 cm lesions that could not be closed primarily over his pre-tibial regions. On one limb, he underwent a fascial release technique (after a vertically orientated elliptical excision) and on the other, a Type 1 keystone design island perforator flap. We did not find any biomechanical advantage in a keystone flap (with its fascia-relaxing incision) when compared with a vertical closure (and a parallel fascia-relaxing incision). There were no wound infections and one case of wound dehiscence was managed by dressings alone and did not need secondary closure.

Table 9.1 Wound tension measurements comparing RSTL/wrinkle lines and vertical lines

No	Age/sex	Diagnosis	Defect diameter (cm)	Tension (N) RSTL/wrinkle lines	Tension (N) BEST lines (vertical)	Relaxing parallel skin incision	Relaxing parallel fascial incision	Variance decrease in tension when using BEST line (vertical closure vs. other directions)	Tension after using parallel relaxing incision	Further decrease in tension when using parallel incision and BEST line closure
1	69/M[a]	BBC	3.5	3.1	2.6		Yes	16.1%	2.4	7.6%
2	69/M[a]	BBC	3.5	3.2	2.8		Keystone	12.5%	2.7	10.7%
3	88/M	SCC	2.7	2.1	1.9		Yes	9.8%	1.7	10.5%
4	79/F	SCC	4	3.2	2.6		Yes	12.5%	2.6	7.1%
5	75/M	BCC	3.5	3.1	2.6		Yes	16.1%	2.4	7.6%
6	87/F	MM wider	4.5	3.1	2.6		Yes	16.1%	2.3	11.5%
7	86/F	SCC	2.0	1.7	1.4	Yes		17.6%	1.3	7.1%
8	75/M[b]	BCC	4.0	3.2	2.8		Yes	12.5%	2.5	10.7%
9	75/M[b]	BCC	3.4 (P)	2.5	2.3		Yes	8%	2.1	8.6%
10	69/F	KA	2.9	1.3	1.1	Yes		15.4%	1.0	9.09%
11	69/M	BCC	4.5	3.6	2.7		Yes	25%	2.4	11.11%
12	80/F	SCC	2.2 (P)	1.5	1.3	Yes		20%	1.2	7.6%
13	88/M	SCC	4.5	3.6	2.7		Yes	25%	2.3	14.81%
14	50/F	BCC	2.0	1.5	1.2	Yes		20%	1.1	8.33%
15	82/M	SCC	3.0	2.4	2.0		Yes	16.7	1.6	20%
16	71/M	BCC	2.4	2.6	2.2		Yes	15.4%	2.0	9.09%
17	57/M	SCC	3.0	2.5	2.3		Yes	8%	2.3	13.04%
18	57/M	SCC	1.5 (P)	1.3	1.1		15.4%	1.0	9.09%	
19	64/F	SCC	2.5	2.3	2.1		Yes	8.7%	2.0	4.7%
20	76/M	SCC	4.0 (P)	3.1	2.6		Yes	16.1%	2.0	23.07%
21	83/F	SCC	3.8	2.4	2.0		Yes	16.7%	1.7	15%

(continued)

Table 9.1 (continued)

No	Age/sex	Diagnosis	Defect diameter (cm)	Tension (N) RSTL/wrinkle lines	Tension (N) BEST lines (vertical)	Relaxing parallel skin incision	Relaxing parallel fascial incision	Variance decrease in tension when using BEST line (vertical closure vs. other directions)	Tension after using parallel relaxing incision	Further decrease in tension when using parallel incision and BEST line closure
22	79/M	SCC	5.0	3.6	2.7		Yes	25%	2.4	11.11%
23	76/M	SCC	2.4	2.6	2.2		Yes	15.4%	2.0	9.09%
								Average reduction in tension 15.82%		Average further reduction in tension 10.71%

The effect of parallel relaxing incisions (with or without fascial release) is noted

[a]Identical lesions on both pretibial regions of this patient. On one side the fascial relaxing incision was used, and on the other a Keystone Design Perforator Island Flap

[b]Lesions were located on both legs of this patient. Some were located posteriorly (P)

Detailed statistical analyses were undertaken at the statistics and mathematics sciences department. The team decided to use the paired t-test (a, b, paired = TRUE). The results are summarized below:

Statistical analyses:

Detailed analysis of skin lines (RSTL vs. BEST) and vertical closure (BEST) vs. vertical closure with a parallel-relaxing incision (PRI) were undertaken by the statistics and mathematical sciences department at the Auckland University of Technology.

Skin Lines RSTL vs. BEST Lines:

Paired t-test, Student's t distribution: $t = 8.9154$, df = 22, $p = 9.338e\text{-}09$. (95% confidence interval): mean of the differences 0.4130435 (41%) showing a statistically significant reduction in wound-closure tension using BEST lines.

BEST vs. BEST + PRI:

Paired t-test, Student's t distribution: $t = 8.7781$, df = 22, $p = 1.223e\text{-}08$. Ninety-five percent confidence interval: mean of the differences 0.2304348 (23%) showing a statistically significant additional reduction in tension when using a parallel-relaxing incision (PRI), also in the vertical plane.

In summary, closure in the vertical direction i.e. orientating the ellipse vertically (Figs. 9.2 and 9.3) showed far less tension than closure along the RSTL/wrinkle

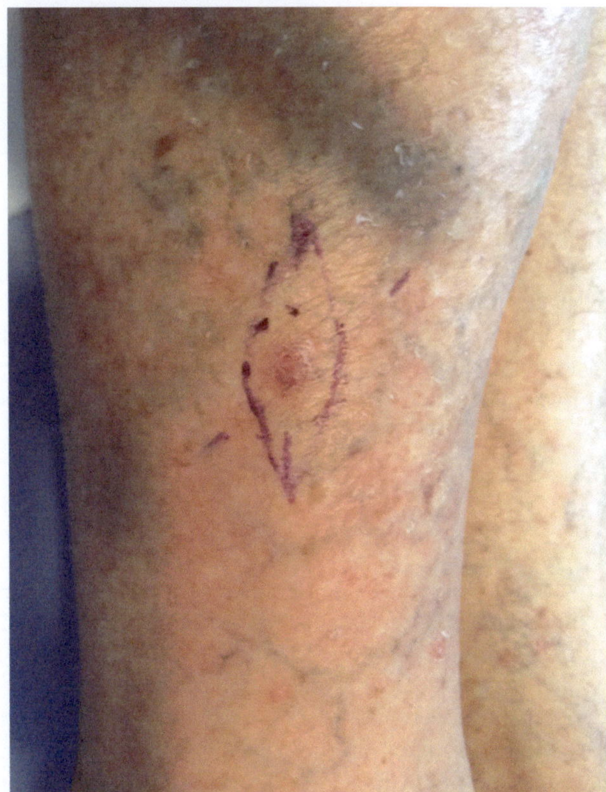

Fig. 9.2 Skin crease lines (RSTL) and incision along vertical (BEST) lines

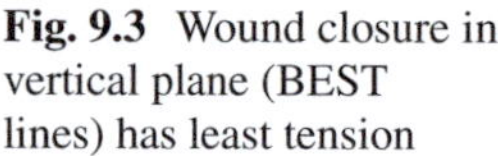

Fig. 9.3 Wound closure in vertical plane (BEST lines) has least tension

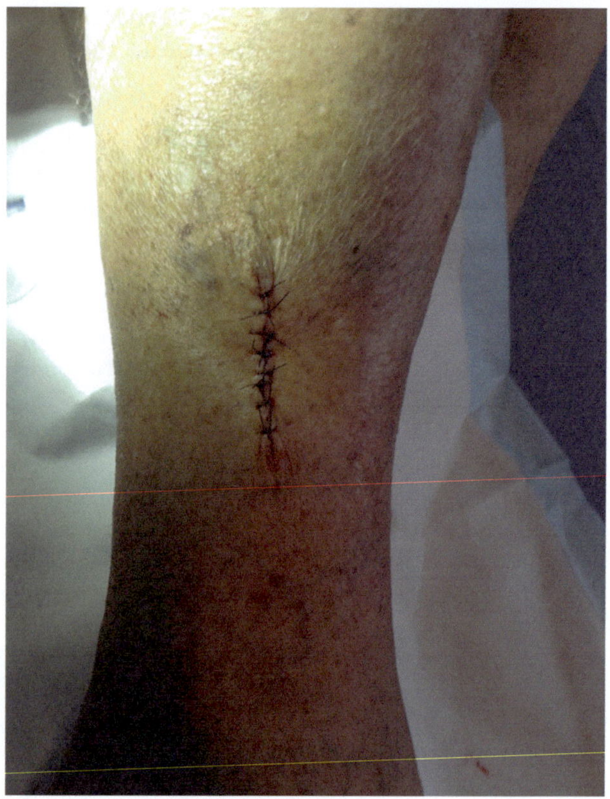

lines of the lower leg, thereby indicating that when it comes to the lower limb, Biodynamic Excisional Skin Tension (BEST) lines (Figs. 9.4 and 9.5) run in the vertical direction. There was no reduction in tension between a keystone design island perforator flap and a vertical parallel incision in the patient who had lesions of similar diameter and wound tension. Using a parallel relaxing incision (Fig. 9.6) further reduced tension by around 10% indicating the usefulness of this technique.

9.4   Discussion

Lower limb, especially below-knee skin cancer excisions pose a problem due to actinic-damaged thin skin that is friable in older patients. When incorrectly oriented ellipses are marked while planning excisions, the end-result is often a skin graft with its associated poor cosmetic appearance. As authors such as Borges have noted, Langer's lines were first studied in cadavers stiffened with rigor mortis so they can hardly be considered lines of relaxation [18]. However, in the lower limb Borges deferred to wrinkle lines [18]. In anatomical locations other than the face, Borges's

Fig. 9.4 BEST lines and wrinkle/RSTL lines leg illustrated in a clinical image

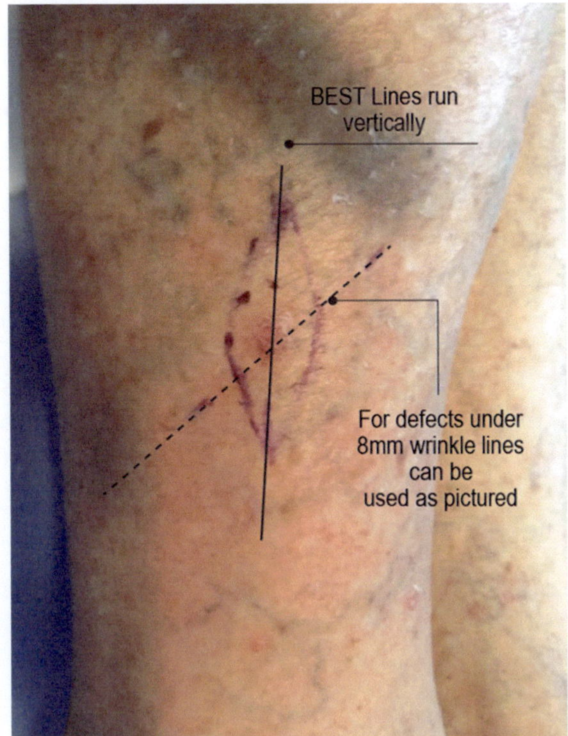

Fig. 9.5 BEST lines, RSTL and location of lesions in this study

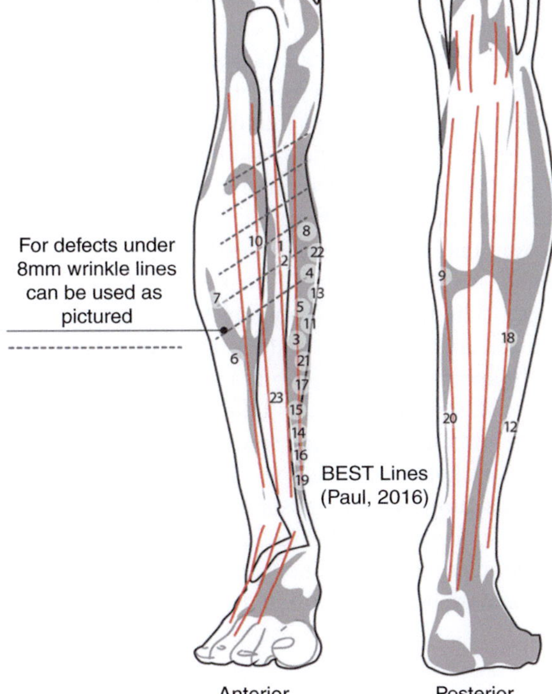

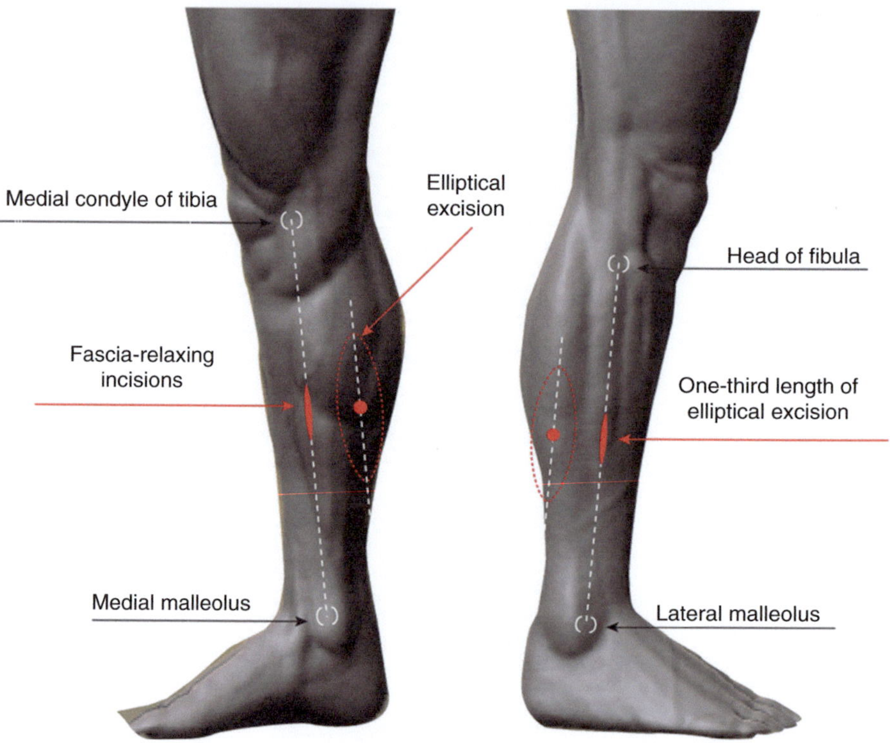

Fig. 9.6 Elliptical excision and parallel relaxing incision technique

lines indeed follow Langer's lines, and in directions against Langer's lines, they are impeded by the skin tension that ends up making them irregular [25]. One of the other problems has been that different textbooks have marked out Langer's lines on the lower limb differently, adding to the confusion during planning excisions [17].

We used Borges method of determining RSTL i.e. pinching skin and noting both furrows and ridges—because when contour lines are produced by muscle of joint action, one only notes furrows [17] and this may be misleading. Using this technique, RSTL and wrinkle lines i.e. skin lines that we observe on our legs at rest seem to lie in the same oblique-horizontal plane (Fig. 9.4). BEST lines for wound closure are noted to be in the vertical plane on the limbs (Fig. 9.2).

In areas like the pre-tibial region of the lower limb, Langer's lines are aligned along elastin fibres—and studies have suggested that 76% of these elastin fibres are in the direction of Langer lines, and 5.1% perpendicular [26]. Another study using a multi-photon microscopic camera has demonstrated that under low-load levels such as during incisional surgery, elastin stretches and collagen buckles, the reverse of what occurs at high-load levels during excisional surgery [27]. Given this differential interplay between elastin and collagen based on low or high loads of tension, the importance of differentiating incisional and excisional lines is important [28], and this may be most important on the lower limb. As this study has shown, biodynamic excisional skin tension (BEST) lines lie in the vertical direction, and are best adopted for lower limb excisional surgery. Additional reduction in tension can be afforded by using parallel relaxing incisions and the details and the surface markings for this specific technique are detailed below.

9.5   Parallel Relaxing Incisions to Decrease Wound Tension

Anatomical studies on vascularity of the lower limb have suggested that the surgical plane lies deep to the fascia layer [1]. Dye-injection studies on cadavers showed that that the fascial plexus communicates with the sub-dermal plexus and sometimes with a vascular plexus on the underside of the deep fascia [1]. Fascial release as an adjunct to wound closure has been described previously, but in the technique advocated by Dumanian, the facial release was performed via the main surgical wound i.e. these fascial releasing incisions resulted in two bi-pedicled fascial flaps attached to the overlying skin [29]. This technique is not dissimilar to the galeal scoring technique that has been used in scalp surgery to reduce wound tension—a method that has been described as "separating components" of skin [30].

The surface markings for the parallel relaxing incisions are as follows (Fig. 9.6): for a medially placed incision the line runs from the medial condyle of tibia to the medial malleolus, and for a laterally placed incision the line runs from the head of the fibula to the lateral malleolus. The site of the relaxing incisions (medial or lateral) is chosen depending on where the lesion is located (anterior or posterior), and the closest location is chosen. In general, the relaxing incision is one-third the length of the ellipse (Fig. 9.6). Care is taken while making the incision through skin and fascia to avoid underlying nerves and blood vessels, and fascia is incised only if the wound is unable to be closed with the parallel relaxing skin incision extending only up to the sub-cutis.

One patient, a 69-year old male, had identical 3.5 cm lesions on both legs and one limb, he underwent a fascial release technique (after vertical excision) and on the other, a Type 1 keystone design island perforator flap. We did not find any biomechanical advantage in a keystone flap (with a fascia-relaxing incision) when compared with a vertical closure (and a parallel fascia-relaxing incision) indicating that the main advantage of the Keystone Flap may not be biomechanics but vascularity. In this case, the parallel relaxing fascial incision actually achieved a greater reduction in tension. As detailed in the table (Table 9.1) above, the use of a parallel relaxing incision reduced tension on vertically closed wounds (on average) by an additional 10.4%. The author noted that pinching the skin (the usual method advocated to find relaxed skin tension lines (RSTL) was often inaccurate indicating that pinching skin may be unreliable on the lower limb to detect best excisional skin tension lines). Wounds that were felt to be too tight to close using the pinch method were easily closed using the parallel relaxing incision technique (Figs. 9.7 and 9.8).

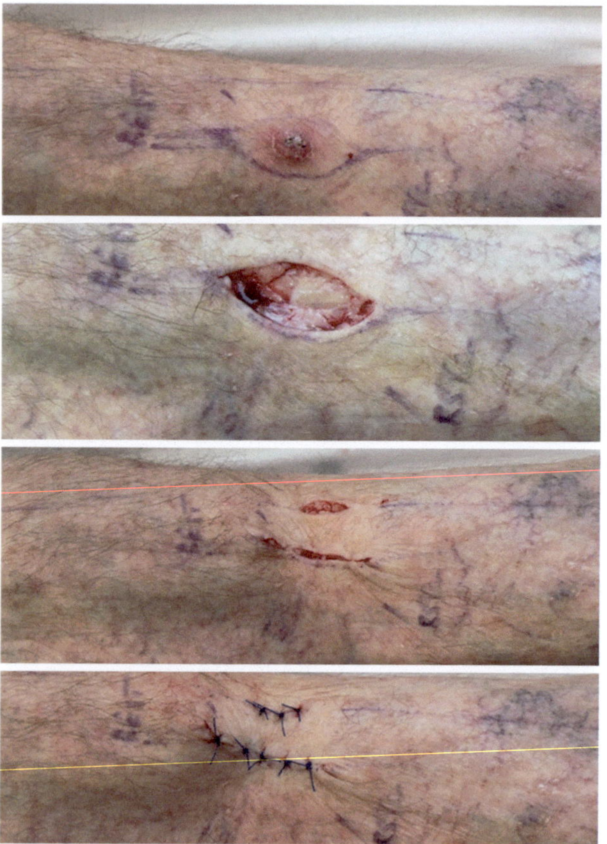

Fig. 9.7 Clinical images of closure using BEST lines and parallel-relaxing incisions

This parallel-relaxing incisional technique has the added advantage of not being limited to a specific site on the leg—as using the surface markings the author has described allows the closure of both anterior and posterior leg wounds. Therefore, this technique is an excellent viable alternative to skin grafts or flap closures for difficult defects. With the surface markings described in this chapter, this author has sometimes used two parallel relaxing incisions for very large closures (Fig. 9.9) or wide excisions.

9.6   Conclusion

This study, that has previously been the subject of another journal article [31] confirms that biodynamic excisional skin tension (BEST) lines that allow the wound to be closed under least tension lie in the vertical direction in the lower limb, and are

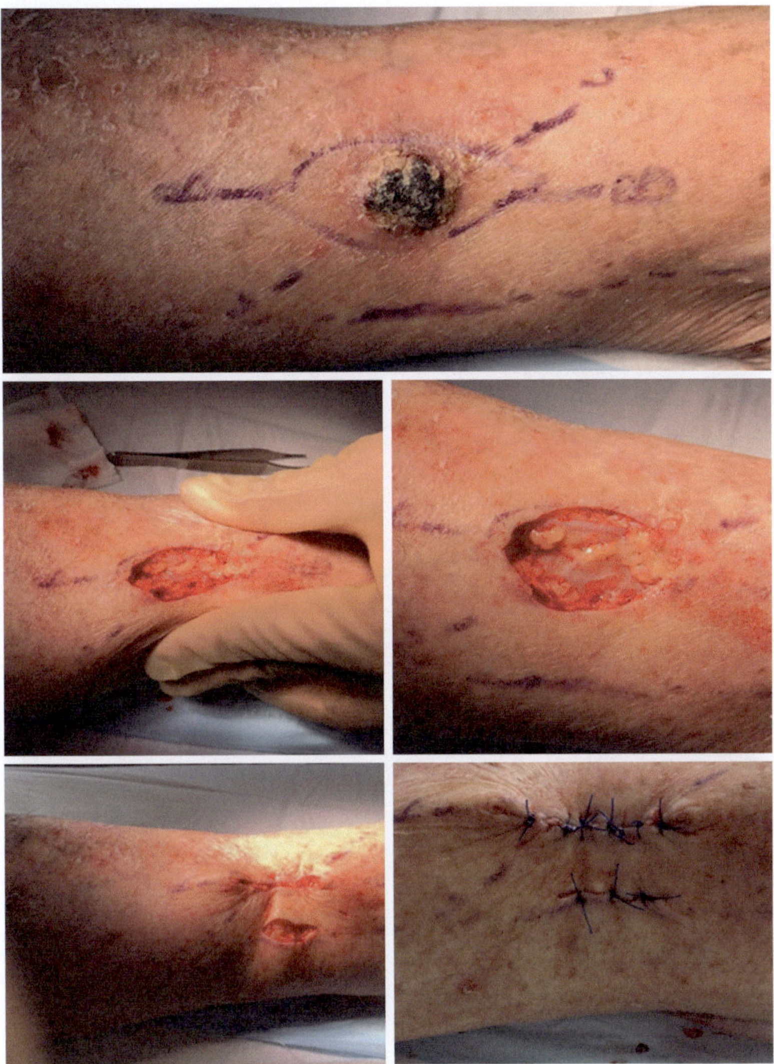

Fig. 9.8 Clinical images of closure using BEST lines and parallel-relaxing incisions. Pinching skin may give an erroneous impression regarding skin tension

best adopted for lower limb excisional surgery. Additional reduction in tension can be achieved by using parallel relaxing incisions, through fascia if needed, also in the vertical plane. The findings of this study suggest that the technique of using parallel relaxing incisions can help achieve the closure of large lower limb defects without utilizing a flap or a skin graft, and is therefore being presented to the wider surgical community [31].

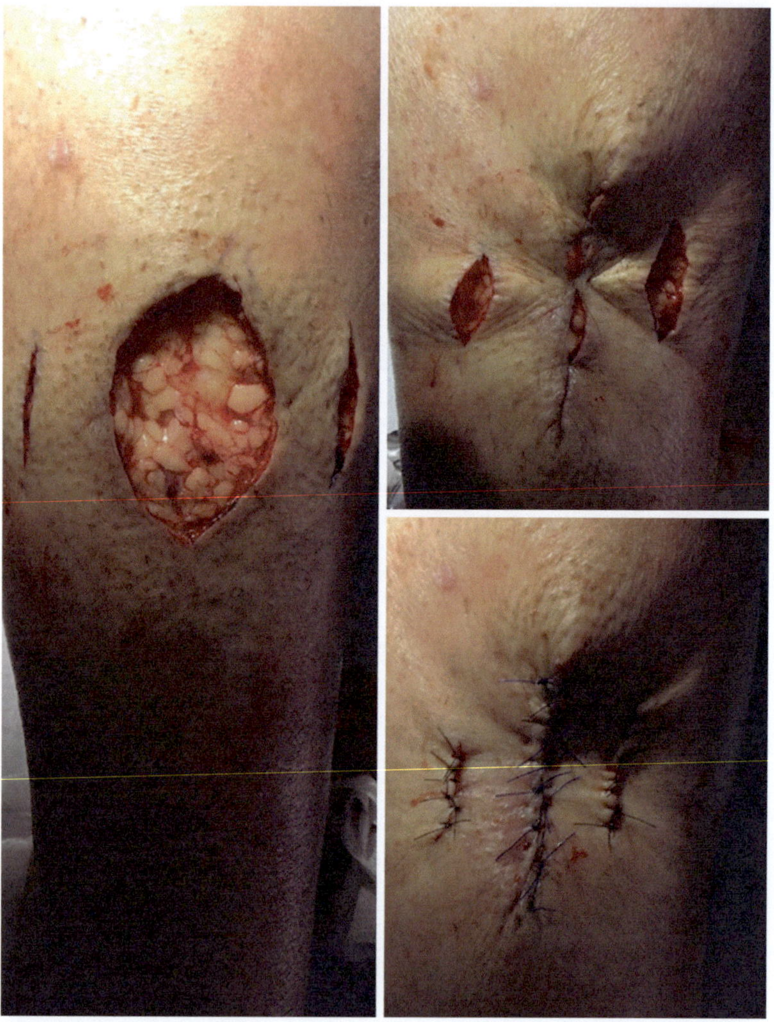

Fig. 9.9 Double parallel relaxing incisions for large calf defects after skin cancer excision

References

1. Haertsch P. The surgical plane in the leg. Br J Plast Surg. 1981;34(4):464–9.
2. Morris CD, Sepkowitz MD, Fonshell C, Margetson N, Eagan J, Miransky J, Boland PJ, Healey J. Prospective identification of risk factors for wound infection after lower extremity oncologic surgery. Ann Surg Oncol. 2003;10:778–82.
3. McNees P. Skin and wound assessment and care in oncology. Semin Oncol Nurs. 2003;22(3):130–43.
4. Dormand E-L, Banwell PE, Goodacre TEE. Radiotherapy and wound healing. Int Wound J. 2005;2:112–27.
5. Schweinberger MH, Roukis YS. Wound complications. Clin Podiatr Med Surg. 2008;26:1–10.

6. Siddiqui A, Bernstein J. Chronic wound infection: facts and controversies. Clin Dermatol. 2010;28:516–26.

7. Shibuya N, Humphers JM, Fluhman BL, Jupiter DC. Factors associated with nonunion, delayed union, and malunion in foot and ankle surgery in diabetic patients. J Foot Ankle Surg. 2013;52:201–11.

8. Goldminz D, Bennett RG. Cigarette smoking and flap and full-thickness graft necrosis. Arch Dermatol. 1991;127:1012.

9. Attinger C, Cooper P, Blume P, Bulan E. The safest surgical incisions and amputations apply the angiosome principles and using Doppler to assess arterial-arterial connections of the foot and ankle. Foot Ankle Clin N Am. 2001;6:745–99.

10. Ueno C, Hunt TK, Hopf HW. Using physiology to improve surgical wound outcomes. Plast Reconstr Surg. 2006;117:59–71S.

11. Parrett BM, Pribaz JJ. Lower extremity reconstruction. Rev Med Clin Condes. 2010;21(1):66–75.

12. Oganesyan G, Jarell AD, Srivastava M, Jiang SI. Efficacy and complication rates of full-thickness skin graft repair of lower extremity wounds after Mohs micrographic surgery. Dermatol Surg. 2013;9(9):1334–9. https://doi.org/10.1111/dsu.12254.

13. Paul SP. "Halo" grafting—a simple and effective technique of skin grafting. Dermatol Surg. 2010;36:115–9. https://doi.org/10.1111/j.1524–4725.2009.01363.x.

14. Behan FC. The keystone design perforator island flap in reconstructive surgery. ANZ J Surg. 2003;73(3):112–20.

15. Dixon AJ, Dixon JB. Reducing opposed multilobed flaps results in fewer complications than traditional repair techniques when closing medium-sized defects on the leg after excision of skin tumor. Dermatol Surg. 2006;32:935–42.

16. Miyamoto S, Kayano S, Fujiki M, Chuman H, Kawai A, Sakuraba M. Early mobilization after free-flap transfer to the lower extremities: preferential use of flow-through anastomosis. Plast Reconstr Surg. 2014;2(3):e127. https://doi.org/10.1097/GOX.0000000000000080.

17. Paul SP. Biodynamic excisional skin tension (BEST) lines: revisiting Langer's lines, skin biomechanics, current concepts in cutaneous surgery, and the (lack of) science behind skin lines used for surgical excisions. J Dermatol Res. 2017;2(1):77–87.

18. Borges AF. Relaxed skin tension lines (RSTL) versus other skin lines. Plast Reconstr Surg. 1984;73(1):144–50.

19. Maranda EL, Heifetz R, Cortizo J, Hafeez F, Nouri K. Kraissl lines—a map. JAMA Dermatol. 2016;152(9):1014. https://doi.org/10.1001/jamadermatol.2016.0325.

20. Paul SP, Matulich N, Charlton N. A new skin tensiometer device: computational analyses to understand biodynamic excisional skin tension lines. Sci Rep. 2016;6:30117. https://doi.org/10.1038/srep30117.

21. Daly CH, Odland GF. Age-related changes in the mechanical properties of human skin. J Invest Dermatol. 1979;73:84–7.

22. Escoffier C, de Rigal J, Rochefort A, Vasselet R, Leveque JL, Agache PG. Age-related mechanical properties of human skin: an in vivo study. J Invest Dermatol. 1989;93(3):353–7.

23. Paul SP. Revisiting Langer's lines, introducing BEST lines, and studying the biomechanics of scalp skin. Spectr Dermatol. 2017;2:8–11.

24. Lanir Y. A structural theory for the homogeneous biaxial stress-strain relationship in flat collageneous tissue. J Biomech. 1979;12:423–36.

25. Barbenel JC. Identification of Langer's lines. In: Serup J, Jemec GBE, editors. Handbook of non-invasive methods and the skin. Boca Raton: CRC Press; 1995. p. 341–4.

26. Zahouani H, Djaghloul M, Vargiolu R, Mezghani S, Mansori MEL. Contribution of human skin topography to the characterization of dynamic skin tension during senescence: morphomechanical approach. J Phys Conf Ser. 2014;483(1):012012.

27. Paul SP. Are incisional and excisional skin tension lines biomechanically different? Understanding the interplay between elastin and collagen during surgical procedures. IJBM. 2017;7(2):111–4.

28. Paul SP. The use of zigs and zags to reduce scarring over "Keloid triangles" during excisional surgery: biomechanics, review and recommendations. Surg Sci. 2017;8:240–55.
29. Dumanian GA, Llull R, Edington H. Fascial release as an adjunct to wound closure. Br J Plast Surg. 1996;49(1):64–6.
30. Ramirez OM, Ruas E, Dellon AL. "Components separation" method for closure of abdominal-wall defects: an anatomic and clinical study. Plast Reconstr Surg. 1990;86:519–26.
31. Paul SP. Biodynamic excisional skin tension (BEST) lines for excisional surgery of the lower limb and the technique of using parallel relaxing incisions to reduce wound tension. Plast Reconstr Surg. 2017;5(12):e1614.

Chapter 10
Understanding Vascular Anatomy of the Lower Limb to Help the Planning of Perforator Based Island Flaps

When considering excisions on the leg, one must appreciate its unique anatomy—subcutaneous bone surrounded by tendons, and vessels in isolated compartments with little intercommunication [1]. Before excision of skin lesions on the leg one must consider the underlying vascularity. And, there are misconceptions—even for free flap transfers, angiograms are rarely needed; in a prospective study of 36 patients, Lutz et al. found that in none of the cases (with at least one palpable pulse) did pre-operative angiography add any valuable information [2]. It is also common after lower limb surgery to advise elevation of the leg. Studies done by Kawasaki and others suggests that the sitting position is equally effective in ensuring a good blood supply to the limb not only in healthy adults, but also in patients with critical limb ischemia [3]. However, allowing lower limbs to hang downwards for long periods time after surgery can cause oedema due to a fall in venous return in lower limbs, and this can result in delayed wound healing [3].

First insights into perforator based flaps emerged when Koshima and others [4] described such flaps on the lower limb. Since then improvement in the anatomical knowledge of cutaneous, subcutaneous, and intramuscular vessels originating from major vascular axis of the limbs has allowed the designing of several types of perforator flaps [5]. The Keystone Design Island Perforator flap, described by Behan [6] has become a very commonly used procedure in Australasia. Panse et al. attempted to correlate the length of such perforator flaps with the length of the limb, and concluded that there was a sixfold increase in flap necrosis if the flap was more than a third of limb-length, as opposed to (if the flap was) less than a third of limb-length [7].

The Gent (Belgium) International Course on Perforator Flaps defines perforator flaps as flaps composed of skin and subcutaneous fat nourished by perforators arising from deep vascular systems, which reach the surface by passing mostly through muscle and intramuscular septa [8]. Anatomically, there is agreement between surgeons and anatomists that a perforator is a vessel that enters the supra-fascial plane through a defined fenestration in the deep fascia [9]. Therefore, perforator flaps can be performed based on any type of perforator. Such "ad hoc perforator flaps"

© Springer International Publishing AG, part of Springer Nature 2018
S. P. Paul, *Biodynamic Excisional Skin Tension Lines for Cutaneous Surgery*,
https://doi.org/10.1007/978-3-319-71495-0_10

relegate the anatomical knowledge and importance of a single flap source vessel as irrelevant, because a flap can be based on any of the 300 or more major perforators that have been described across the body [10]. In this context, Taylor and Palmer have done valuable work in mapping perforators [10].

One cannot consider biodynamic excisional skin tension (BEST) lines for cutaneous surgery on the lower limb without commenting on blood supply—and therefore this chapter seeks to understand the vascular anatomy of the lower limb.

10.1   Introduction to Lower Limb Perforators

Reconstruction of the lower leg after skin cancer excisions can be challenging due to actinic damaged thinned-out skin that is friable, and poor vascularity in patients with diabetes or other diseases that impact the vascular system. Even in healthy individuals, the lower limb presents a specific challenge due to the "surgical plane" of the lower limb. When it comes to closing large defects on the lower limb, random pattern cutaneous flaps are also limited by the arc of rotation and a resulting decrease in bacterial resistance, and a generally accepted rule of a 2:1 ratio between the length and base of the flap [11].

Skin flaps, especially random cutaneous flaps have fared poorly on the lower limb and probably because, as literature reviews have shown, most flaps have been raised superficial to the deep fascia [12]. Haertsch conducted a dye-injection study on 22 post-mortem legs and demonstrated the role of the fascial plexus. His study showed that the fascial plexus communicated with the sub-dermal plexus, and sometimes with a vascular plexus on the undersurface of the deep fascia. Haertsch confirmed, that for practical purposes, the 'surgical plane' of the leg lies deep to the deep fascia [12].

Given this "surgical plane" of the lower limb, many surgeons have designed perforator-based flaps and have used Doppler probes to try and incorporate perforators into the base of a flap [13]. While the hand-held Doppler device has often been used to identify perforators in the lower limb, review of the literature suggests that that most of such unidirectional Doppler flowmetry analyses for perforator-based flaps have been done predominantly on the trunk [13]. Authors have noted that while a handheld Doppler can demonstrate the direction of blood flow, it fails to determine the size of the vessel or its flow volume—thereby resulting in high false-positive (or false-negative results) at extremities like the lower limb [3]. Using a colour Doppler can obviate some of these risks, but all Doppler devices are very operator dependent—both in terms of skill, and prior anatomical knowledge of perforator locations [13].

Given the variability of lower limb perforators and the difficulty in identifying specifics islands of tissue that can be perfused by reliably-identifiable perforators, recent studies have attempted to use CT scans to study locations of perforators—with authors noting that CT angiography was able to show perforators with high resolution and accurately demonstrate vessel size, location and course [14]. It is now established that in almost all cases, distal arterial perforators have veins accompanying them. In general, a vein lies inferior to the artery and when there are two veins, they often tend to interconnect around the artery.

While island flaps such as the V-Y advancement island flap, the Bezier flap and the Keystone Design Island flap are often mentioned in the context of perforator-based island flaps of the lower limb, one issue with conventional island flaps is that when tissue is advanced or transposed, a twist of tissue occurs and this increases the external pressure on the venous supply. It is a well-known plastic surgical dictum that fascio-cutaneous flaps, once "islanded," are solely reliant on the venae commitantes for venous drainage. Therefore, it is important to know where reliable venous perforator drainage exists, as this can help plan the location of such islands. The author therefore set out to study lower limbs using a thermal imaging camera to see if we could find reliable perforator locations in the lower limbs that could help in the design of perforator-based fascio-cutaneous flaps.

10.2 Materials and Methods

In this study, a thermal imaging camera (FLIR®One for iPhone, manufactured by Flir Systems Inc.) was used to take images of lower limbs prior to cutaneous surgery (planning island flaps). This device contains a non-contact spot temperature measurement with automatic shuttering, and has been designed to capture a thermal reading of photographic images—and therefore in the past, has been primarily used in detecting leaks in buildings.

The protocol for this study and informed consent were approved by an institutional review board, in our case the HDECS Ethics Approval Committee, and all subjects gave informed consent: all ethics approvals were approved by the relevant authorities—New Zealand: Health and Disability Ethics Committee (HDEC Reference number 15/CEN/113); Australia: Queensland Institutional Human Ethics (Approval No. 2015001550).

A total of 23 cases formed part of this study—16 were pretibial lesions, 4 were located closer to the ankle and 3 were located on the calf. We found the use of thermal imaging camera technically easy and with insignificant user-variation. It was easy to identify thermal patterns for venous perfusion (whiteness) and arterial suffusion (redness) as noted in a case where a fasciotomy had been performed (Fig. 10.1). What was immediately apparent was the remarkable consistency of venous perforator "islands" on the lower limb—we noted them in three particular locations that corresponded with previously noted locations of perforator clusters in the lower limb.

We marked out the regions proximally from the inter-malleolar line. Venous perforators were shown to be concentrated in certain segments (Fig. 10.2). The first cluster was at 5–10 cm from the inter-malleolar line that corresponded with known locations of anterior tibial artery perforators that originate between the tibia and tibialis anterior muscle. Anteriorly, the main larger cluster was at 20–25 cm

Fig. 10.1 Thermal imaging: increased arterial perfusion (redness) after a fasciotomy

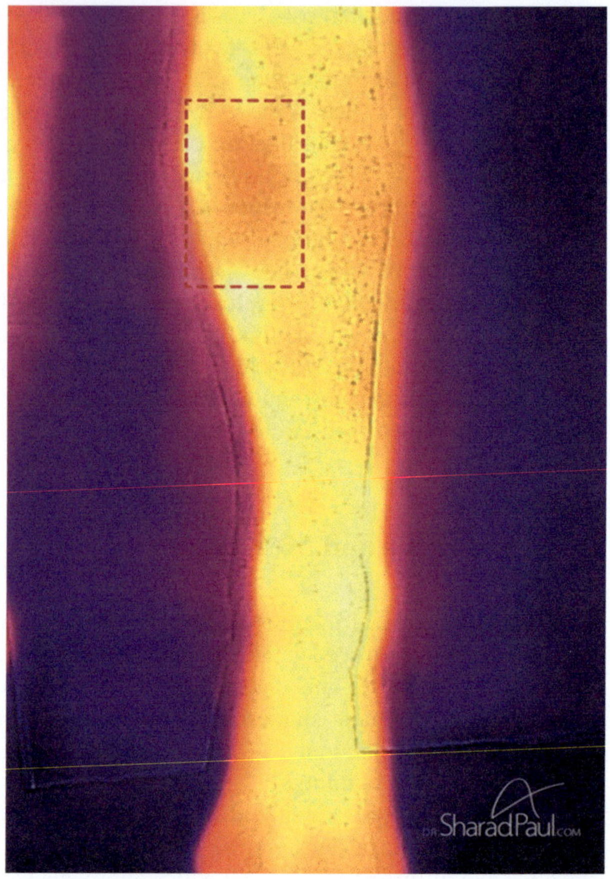

proximal to this inter-malleolar line, and this corresponds with perforators that originate via the anterior peroneal septum, between the extensor digitorum longus and the peroneus longus muscles (Fig. 10.2). Posteriorly on the calf, there was a cluster at 13–18 cm—corresponding with known perforators from the peroneal artery that course through the posterior peroneal septum as indicated in the image (Fig. 10.3).

We must note that in using this technique—as while using handheld Dopplers or ultrasound, there is some degree of operator experience required, especially knowledge of the optimum imaging distance, in order to achieve consistent and reproducible results. The idea here was to mark out "perforator islands" as a guide for cutaneous surgery. We essentially mapped locations of blocks of tissue with adequate venous perfusion that can be utilized for island flaps. We did not set out to identify specific perforators, which we believe is not achievable consistently. However, as noted in the image (Fig. 10.4) others have successfully used this thermal imaging technique to raise island flaps such as the Bezier Island flap—even managing to incorporate a specific venous perforator.

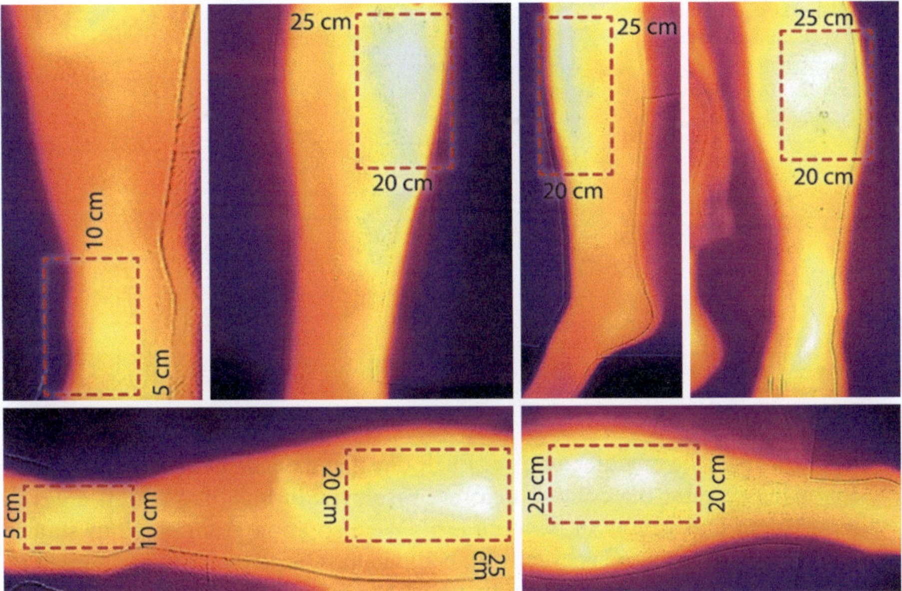

Fig. 10.2 Anterior tibial artery perforators: Perforators from Anterior tibial artery are in two distinct segments, most prominent 20–25 cm from inter-malleolar line (whiteness indicates venous perfusion)

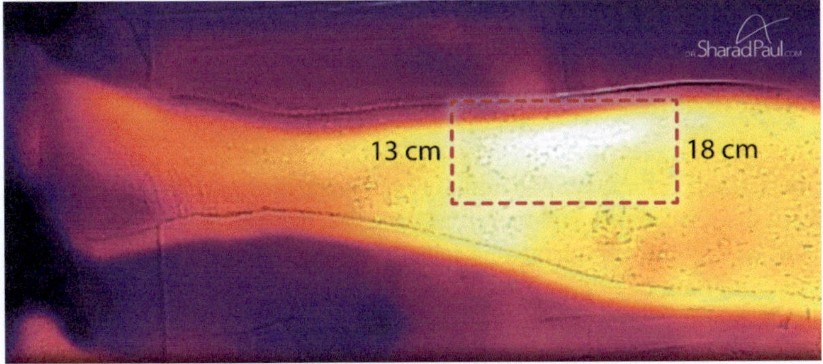

Fig. 10.3 Peroneal artery perforators. Posteriorly calf perforators from the peroneal artery are located at a cluster 13–18 cm from the inter-malleolar line

The technique for using the FLIR®One Camera to identify venous perforators has already been defined. Suphachokauychai and others have already provided guidelines for the use of these cameras to obtain accurate results [15]. They noted that firstly the camera should be used on a dry surface. Ideally the measuring distance is around the 100 cm mark, and the thermal range should be locked at 25–30 °C. Those authors note that this technique has become their favoured one for identifying vascular perforators, allowing them the freedom to design a freestyle perforator flap [15].

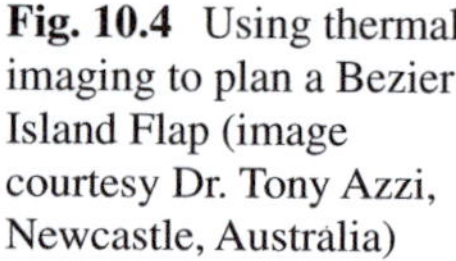

Fig. 10.4 Using thermal imaging to plan a Bezier Island Flap (image courtesy Dr. Tony Azzi, Newcastle, Australia)

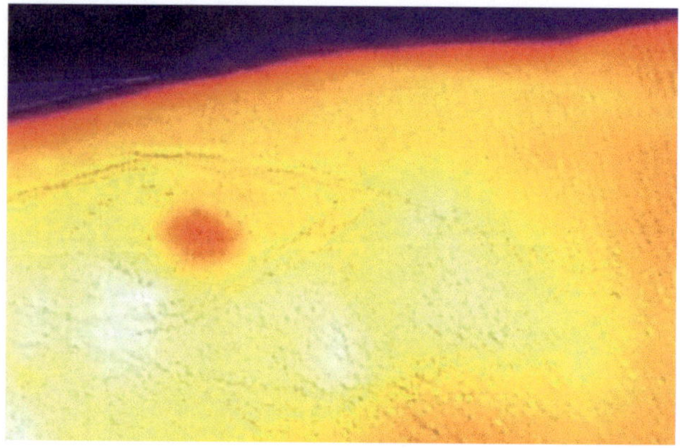

We know from the manufacturers of FLIR one that the palette of colours exhibits the following pattern: the coldest areas are displayed in blue, the hottest areas in white, with red and yellow in between [16]. We also know from previous studies that the venous temperature is usually higher than the temperature in the artery [17]. And when it comes to tumours, or rather heat conduction through surrounding tissue—tumour heat reaches the skin surface or is transported indirectly via venous blood flow to the skin [17]. Given venous perforators are hotter than arteries in the legs, we expected the veins to display a whitish palette and this was what we noted in this study.

10.3   Discussion

As we have noted earlier, venous drainage plays a major part in ensuring island flap viability in the lower limb, and therefore there is a need to identify locations of suitable blood supply—from whence an island flap can be mobilized. Detailed cadaveric dissections have been done by others [15], who also noted that major perforators of the lower leg were located in three similar distinct clusters.

In summary, the lower limb has three main clusters of perforating veins (Fig. 10.5) that are especially useful in designing island fascio-cutaneous flaps, as venous drainage can be the defining criterion for viability of these flaps. We undertook a literature review of cadaveric dissections that had previously identified known perforator locations after our study was completed, and were pleasantly surprised to note that our findings correlated very closely with the results noted by Schaverien and colleagues [18]. These correspond with locations where island perforator flaps are generally more successful. In the illustration (Fig. 10.6) the authors noted that perforators are found between the flexor digitorum longus and soleus at three intervals, with the largest perforators found in the middle cluster (center image). Illustration of the lower leg after cadaveric dissections shows the location of reliable perforators from the anterior tibial artery, the proximal cluster, from 21 to 25 cm,

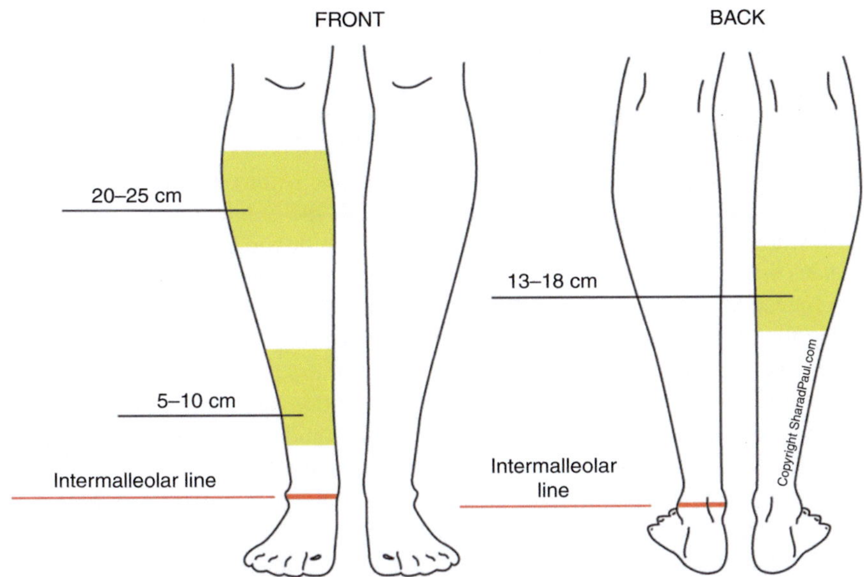

Fig. 10.5 Venous 'islands' of the lower limb. The lower limb has three main clusters of perforating veins that are especially useful in designing island fascio-cutaneous flaps

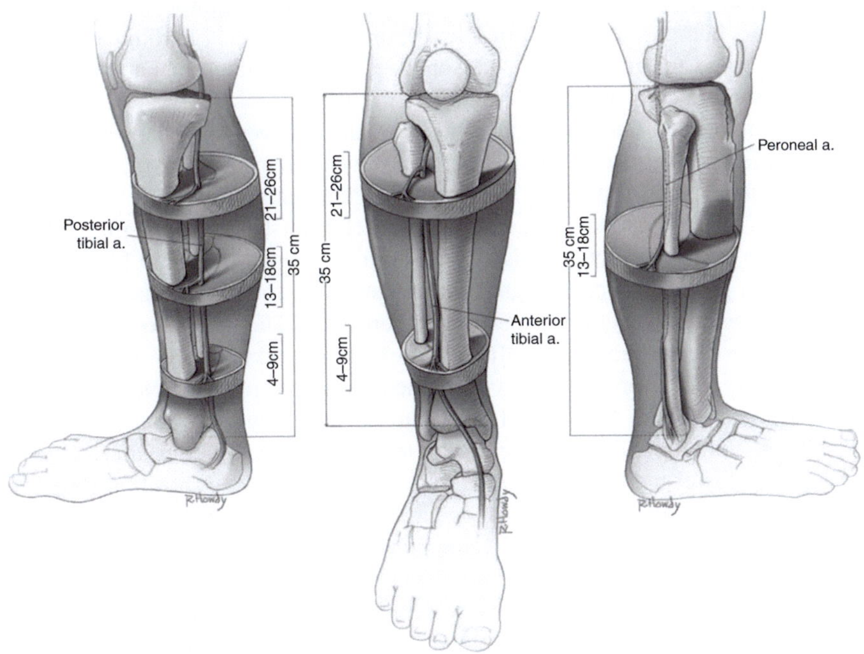

Fig. 10.6 Illustration of the lower leg revealing the location of reliable perforators from the posterior tibial artery (reprinted with permission from Wolters Kluwer; taken from Schaverien M, Saint-Cyr M. Perforators of the lower leg: analysis of perforator locations and clinical application for pedicled perforator flaps. Plast Reconstr Surg. 2008; 122(1):161–70)

that is found within the anterior peroneal septum between the extensor digitorum longus and the peroneus longus. The distal cluster, from 4 to 9 cm, was found between the tibia and the tendon of the tibialis anterior muscle (right image). The illustration of the lower leg also reveals the location of reliable perforators from the peroneal artery.

Another cluster is found between 13 and 18 cm, within the posterior peroneal septum. Proximally, perforators emerged through the soleus or peroneus longus muscles, and distally they were found between the flexor hallucis longus and the peroneus brevis. As illustrated in Figs. 10.2 and 10.3, our study using thermal imaging achieved a remarkable correlation with these cadaver dissection studies demonstrating the usefulness and validity of this technique.

We have presented our method of using thermal imaging to identify perforators in a previous article [19] as that was the first time this had been used in this manner—and this can greatly help in the planning of island flaps. Further, while previous researchers have had to undertake cadaveric dissections, Doppler imaging or CT scans to locate perforators, this technique is simple, performed easily before and during surgery, and is reliably reproducible by different operators. In contrast, Doppler techniques have been noted to have a 45% chance of producing a false positive overall, with the error-rate highest amongst inexperienced surgeons [20]. The thermal imaging camera is therefore more cost effective and being a visual method, more efficient.

The other advantage with this method is that, given some minor individual variations (clusters being more medial or lateral), this author was able to locate perforator clusters prior to surgery and "personalize" surgical flaps in patients. Milton noted in his studies on island flaps that when a flap is "islanded" it is the venous supply that matters [6] and he famously wrote about lower limb flaps saying, "An island is safer than a peninsula" [21]. The ability to map the general locations of perforator islands is of great help in lower limb cutaneous surgery.

As others have concluded, circulation in a perforator-based flap is more physiological when compared with a distally-based axial vessel-type flap [11], and the presence of a positive Doppler signal (or whiteness on thermal imaging, using our method) allows the execution of perforator flaps [22]. The use of local perforator-based flaps for reconstruction of soft tissue defects after skin cancer is a simple and safe alternative to the more complex and time-consuming microsurgical procedures [22]. Flaps such as the Keystone Island flap have merely confirmed what others have noted—that a local fascial flap of the leg can provide a better alternative to a free flap with fewer medical complications, shorter operative or hospital times, and better aesthetic results [23]. Knowledge gained in this chapter should help the planning and design of island perforator flaps. The author would like to add that following studies on BEST lines of the lower limb (detailed in the previous chapter)—using parallel relaxing incisions (with or without incorporation of fascia) is an often better alternative to island flap closure, and offers a better reduction in wound tension—even if a perforator-based island flap may sometimes be necessary to cover bare-bone defects.

References

1. Bajantri B, Bharathi RR, Sabapathy SR. Wound coverage considerations for defects of the lower third of the leg. Indian J Plast Surg. 2012;45(2):283–90.
2. Lutz BS, Wei FC, Machens HG, Rhode U, Berger A. Indications and limitations of angiography before free-flap transplantation to the distal lower leg after trauma: prospective study in 36 patients. J Reconstr Microsurg. 2000;16(3):187–91.
3. Yasir M, et al. Perforator flaps for reconstruction of lower limb defects. Int Surg J. 2016;3(4):2109–14.
4. Koshima I, Moriguchi T, Ohta S. The vasculature and clinical application of the posterior tibial perforator-based flap. Plast Reconstr Surg. 1992;90:643–9.
5. Taylor GI. The angiosomes of the body and their supply to perforator flaps. Clin Plast Surg. 2003;30:331–42.
6. Behan FC. The keystone design perforator island flap in reconstructive surgery. ANZ J Surg. 2003;73:112–20.
7. Panse NS, Bhatt YC, Tandale MS. What is safe limit of the perforator flap in lower extremity reconstruction? Do we have answers yet? Plast Surg Int. 2011;2011:349–57.
8. Horlock N, Pirayesh A, Teo T. The propeller flap: an elegant refinement to the reverse flow fasciocutaneous flap in distal lower limb reconstruction. Presented at the Fifth International Course on Perforator Flaps, Gent. Belgium. Sept 2001:28.
9. Niranjan NS, Price RD, Govilkar P. Fascial feeder and perforator-based V-Y advancement flaps in the reconstruction of lower limb defects. Br J Plast Surg. 2000;53(8):679–89.
10. Taylor GI, Palmer JH. The vascular territories (angiosomes) of the body: experimental study and clinical applications. Br J Plast Surg. 1987;40(2):113–41.
11. Jordan DJ, Malahias M, Hindocha S, Juma A. Flap decisions and options in soft tissue coverage of the lower limb. Open Orthop J. 2014;8:423–32.
12. Haertsch PA. The surgical plane in the leg. Br J Plast Surg. 1981;34:464–9.
13. Khan UD, Miller JG. Reliability of handheld Doppler in planning local perforator–based flaps for extremities. Aesthet Plast Surg. 2007;31(5):521.
14. Ribuffo D, Atzeni M, Saba L, et al. Clinical study of peroneal artery perforators with computed tomographic angiography: implications for fibular flap harvest. Surg Radiol Anat. 2010;32(4):329–34.
15. Suphachokauychai S, Kiranantawat K, Sananpanich K. Detection of perforators using smartphone thermal imaging. JPRAS Glob Open. 2016;4(5):e722. https://doi.org/10.1097/GOX.00000000000000071.
16. FLIR ONE. Technical note. http://www.flir.com/uploadedFiles/Thermography/MMC/Brochures/ T820340/T820340_EN.pdf. Accessed 15 Feb 2017.
17. Lawson RN, Gaston JP. Temperature measurements of localized pathological processes. Ann N Y Acad Sci. 1964;121:90.
18. Schaverien M, Saint-Cyr M. Perforators of the lower leg: analysis of perforator locations and clinical application for pedicled perforator flaps. Plast Reconstr Surg. 2008;122(1):161–70.
19. Paul SP. Using a thermal imaging camera to locate perforators on the lower limb. Arch Plast Surg. 2017;44(3):243–7.
20. Stekelenburg CM, Sonneveld PM, Bouman MB, et al. The hand held Doppler device for the detection of perforators in reconstructive surgery: what you hear is not always what you get. Burns. 2014;40:1702–6.
21. Milton SH. Experimental studies on island flaps. 1. The surviving length. Plast Reconstr Surg. 1971;48(6):574–8.
22. Quaba O, Quaba A. Pedicled perforator flaps for the lower limb. Semin Plast Surg. 2006;20(2):103–11.
23. Bhatti A, Adeshola A, Ismael T, Harris N. Lower leg flaps comparison between free versus local flaps. The Internet. J Plast Surg. 2006;3(2):1–8.

Chapter 11
Anatomical Considerations During Cutaneous Surgery on the Face: Skin Biodynamics, Neurovascular Zones and BEST Lines

When a defect is small, it can be closed primarily and larger defects may need flaps or skin grafts. However, it is often difficult to reproduce the delicate three-dimensional character—caused by the multiple aesthetic units of the face, using a single flap [1]. The hairlines at the forehead and temporal regions and the hair-bearing regions of the upper lip are also important considerations; as is the orientation of excision with respect to the eyelid margin—as any tension can result in delayed ectropion formation much after the surgical excision has been completed.

One way to minimize visible scarring or contour deformity is to treat the central units of the face (within the visual field of the observer) different to the peripheral units—those outside the visual gaze of a person standing in front of the patient. Menick wrote that the subunit principle must be applied to central convex subunits (areas seen during primary gaze that demand contralateral symmetry between the normal and reconstructed side) when using skin flaps [1]. There is another important dictum in plastic surgery to keep in mind when planning reconstruction of these facial units—flaps pincushion; grafts do not.

Closure of an ellipse is the most commonly used excision method for skin cancer [2]. The geometrical shape of the surgical ellipse is derived from the Greek "ellipsis" where the distance between two loci are constant around an orbit, allowing for equalization of wound tension. However, as many have pointed out, a surgical ellipse should be more accurately called a "fusiform excision" because the ends are pointed, rather than rounded [3]. Tapering the ellipse into 30° pointed angles allows one to reduce the appearance of dog-ears. The elliptical excision is an adaptable and easy surgical strategy. When adequate tissue is present for primary closure, a variant of the "tangent-to-circle" approach usually allows the surgeon to orient the suture line within relaxed tension lines [3].

Skin is our largest organ and the only universal organ across animal species [4]. Skin is subject to mechanical-loading during excisional surgery and can double its area when subject to mechanical stretch [5]. In plastic and dermatologic surgery, we not only use this knowledge during excisional surgery, but we also use this knowledge in tissue expansion to achieve better skin coverage by the controlled application

© Springer International Publishing AG, part of Springer Nature 2018
S. P. Paul, *Biodynamic Excisional Skin Tension Lines for Cutaneous Surgery*,
https://doi.org/10.1007/978-3-319-71495-0_11

of stretch [6]. Biomechanical studies have noted the importance of the basement membrane and the mechanical continuity at the basement membrane for optimal force transfer between the epidermis and the dermis [6]. The dermis is 0.5–5.0 mm in thickness, and is the load-bearing inner layer. Of its remaining dry weight (beyond the water content) 80–85% of the dermis consists of loosely interwoven, wavy, randomly-oriented collagen fibres, supplemented by 2–4% of elastin fibres [7]. As we will discuss further in this chapter, skin thickness varies across the face and is important to take this into account while trying to achieve the best cosmetic result by choosing donor sites of similar thickness for flaps and grafts. The biodynamics and mechanical forces that deform skin, or cause stretch have other biological effects that are often underappreciated—as studies have focused only on the physics, and not the physiology of skin stretch [8]. In focusing on the skin, one must not ignore the subcutis because unlike the epidermis and the dermis, the subcutaneous tissue changes upon tissue expansion, and adipocytes become compressed and diminished in size [9]. However, where there is not a lot of subcutaneous fat on the face, the thickness of the epidermal and dermal layers does not change when skin is subjected to stretch [6]. However, on the cheek we need to take heed of both underlying fat, and the neurovascular anatomy—both of which will be discussed in this chapter.

11.1   The History of Skin Line Research on the Face and RSTL

The investigation into surgical lines of the face can be divided into three different methodologies—the study of skin orthotropy employed by Langer and Cox who studied skin cleavage lines, the visual approach favoured by Kraissl and Rubin, and the method of external force such as the pinch technique employed by Borges.

11.1.1   Cleavage Lines of Skin

In 1861 Karl Langer of Vienna began his seminal study into skin lines by puncturing holes in cadavers and noting that the clefts deformed into oval shaped defects. He connected these longitudinal lines and called these "cleavage lines of skin" or "Spaltbarkeit der Cutis" [10]. Langer mapped these cleavage lines but it was not until the end of the century that they ended up as *de facto* surgical lines due to the recommendations of Kocher, a Swiss surgeon [11]. It must be noted that Kocher used these lines for surgical incisions, and did not mention excisions.

In 1938, American surgeon Herbert Conway, MD, noted widening in the lower portion of abdominal scars where excisions were made using Langer's lines concluded that cadaveric skin findings could not be readily applied to living skin with respect to skin tension lines [12]. This led to others looking to repeat Langer's experiments and for other options.

In 1941, Cox from Manchester, decided to repeat Langer's experiment, again in (in this study 28 unclaimed) cadavers. The instrument Cox selected to pierce the skin was a metal-pointed wooden marlinspike and the part that entered the skin resembled the end of a sharply pointed pencil according to Cox's writings [13]. Cox examined approximately 22,600 puncture wounds made using this method and was convinced at the existence of cleavage lines. He noted that these skin line patterns showed variations according to body i.e. muscular or slim build—and was not constant across body types. Cox also commented that Langer's diagrams showed variations according to age. However, Cox felt that it was the shape of the body—rather than its years, that mattered.

Given this variability it made no sense to use these lines universally as excisional lines, although Cox didn't make any comment in this regard. However, Cox wrote: "Skin incisions are followed by skin retraction, the amount of retraction being a measure of the amount of tension. Retraction has been found to be minimal in incisions in the cleavage lines and maximal in incisions made at right angles to these lines. This affords conclusive proof that cleavage lines are lines of increased tension" [13]. On the face, this retraction has been found to be minimal in incisions along these cleavage lines, and maximal in incisions made at right angles to these lines.

11.1.2   Visual Lines of Skin

Cornelius Kraissl took photographs of people after making them contract muscles of facial expression. After comparing many images, he created composite images of wrinkle lines [14]. In areas like the forehead and cheek, wrinkle lines run perpendicular to muscle fibres. However, Kraissl's method created some confusion—as certain expressions like laughing or whistling produce lines in the same areas of the face—but these lines often end up at right angles to each other.

Kraissl and Conway did consider the use of wrinkle lines in the context of skin excisions of "small" tumours of the face [15]. In most cases, wrinkle lines were found to be at right angles to the pull of the muscles. But sometimes strong muscle actions can also cause well developed folds. The risorius and buccinator are especially involved in the defining of the nasolabial groove. Kraissl and Conway felt that wrinkle lines were caused by muscle-shortening without any associated skin-shortening [15]. Skin adapts by forming folds that are at right angles to the actions of underlying muscles on the face. A notable exception being the infraorbital region—where wrinkles are in the direction of the fibres of the orbicularis oculi, and this is important to note in surgical excisions around the eyelids.

Rubin studied skin lines by taking impressions on paper similar to the technique used for finger-printing [16]. A pad was applied to the face, gently coating it with a chemical. When sensitized paper was then applied, it marked the elevated ridges and like Kraissl, Rubin noted that these ridge-lines were in general at right angles to muscle fibres.

11.1.3   Relaxed Skin Tension Lines

Alberto Borges who first described relaxed skin tension lines (RSTL) noted that these were not necessarily visible to the naked eye, but became apparent on pinching skin. He noted that these lines follow furrows when skin is relaxed [17]. As Borges noted, the ridges and furrows formed by pinching skin extend for a greater distance when skin is pinched at right angles to resting skin tension lines and these lines follow the same direction on either side of the pinch. This technique was reliable because there was no specific number of lines—ridges or furrows that needed to be noted; only the general direction these pointed towards. These RSTL exerted a constant force even during sleep, and muscle contractions only caused a temporary disturbance. Borges mapped out the RSTL on the face; however, for the rest of the body he deferred to wrinkle lines as the lines to use for excisions. However, the face, because the SMAS layer has special considerations—and therefore RSTL end up as BEST lines in this location.

11.2   Superficial Musculo-Aponeurotic System (SMAS) of the Face

Animals other than humans have a subdermal system of muscle that allows them to flick off insects and even contract wounds. This panniculus carnosus which is a part of the subcutaneous tissues is a layer of striated muscle deep to the panniculus adiposus [18]—and in human bodies, vestiges of these muscles appear as the platysma in the neck, or the dartos in the scrotum.

In 1976, a landmark paper by Mitz and Peyronie described the superficial musculo-aponeurotic system of the face [19]. These authors described the superficial musculoaponeurotic system (SMAS) in the parotid and cheek regions of the face, and noted that it appeared to divide fat into superficial and deep adipose tissue. The concept of SMAS has since been a regular part of the lexicon of plastic and aesthetic surgery, with numerous anatomical and dissection findings described. In 2010, Macchi and colleagues undertook a cadaveric histotopographic study of the SMAS and confirmed the presence of a laminar connective tissue layer (SMAS) that enclosed two different fibroadipose connective tissue compartments—superficial and deep [20]. The superficial fibroadipose layer presented vertically oriented fibrous septa, connecting the dermis with the superficial aspect of the SMAS; in the deep fibroadipose connective layer, the fibrous septa were obliquely oriented, connecting the deep aspect of the SMAS to the parotid-masseteric fascia [20]. Macchi's team noted that the superficial SMAS thinned out from the pre-auricular region medially towards the nose. In the pre-auricular region, the mean thicknesses of the superficial and deep fibroadipose connective tissues were 1.63 and 0.8 mm, respectively, whereas in the region of the nasolabial fold the superficial layer is not recognizable, while the mean thickness of the deep fibroadipose connective layer was 2.9 mm [20].

Broughton and others undertook further cadaveric dissections to verify Macchi's findings and found the following applied to the anatomy of the SMAS: the SMAS had a layered morphology; it progressively changes from being fibrous to aponeurotic; it envelopes the zygomaticus musculature; regionally, it is seen in temporal but not nasal or forehead regions. The presence of the SMAS in the cervical platysma region remains inconclusive anatomically. However, variability within the platysma muscle influences the extent and thickness of the SMAS layer [21].

Dissecting the SMAS has become well established in aesthetic procedures such as facelifts, and also when large flaps are mobilized to cover defects caused by skin cancer. The lifting and plicating of the SMAS has been traditionally considered essential to achieve better and long-lasting results in face and neck lift procedures, and therefore some authors have modified the original SMAS concept, and renamed it as the SMAFS (superficial musculo-aponeurotic-fatty system) [22]. Such a view considers the superficial muscles of facial expression, the fibro-aponeurotic sheath encircling the muscles, and the superficial fat as a single anatomical unit [22]. Khawaja and others have described several variations in the lower portion of the SMAFS. A breakdown of SMAFS has also been noticed as the result of repeated steroid injections into the face, and a fatty SMAFS is noted in obese patients and those with prominent cheeks. There are also considerable variations of the frontal and marginal mandibular nerves in relation to the SMAFS and this must be carefully noted during surgery [22].

Given this book's focus is on skin tension and biomechanics, it is worth mentioning the mechanical properties of the SMAS layer. Mechanical and microscopic studies have revealed that the SMAS consists of collagen fibres, with a relatively high concentration of elastin fibres interspersed with fat cells. On scanning electron microscopy, the collagen within the virginal SMAS shows a similar convoluted appearance as usually noted in the dermis [23]. Both dermis and SMAS consist of interwoven coiled collagen fibres and the elastin is densely packed to form a fibrous "mat" which is generally not isotropic [23]. The SMAS is lubricated by a viscous mucopolysaccharide extracellular matrix that reduces friction during movements of separate fibres—but imparts a viscous resistance to relative motion and this may explain why on the face RSTL lines contradict wrinkle lines in many areas. This mechanical response of the dermis and SMAS to loading is time-dependent, making the SMAS a viscoelastic material [23]. These coiled interwoven fibres stiffen under stress, making this elastic and fully reversible response highly non-linear.

During surgery, there is a difference between the response to stretch of the SMAS to that of normal skin. Intraoperative stretching of the facial skin over a 40- to 45-min period does cause some slackening [24]. However, when the SMAS is subjected to a similar stretching force to that of the overlying skin, it does not show any evidence of slackening intraoperatively [24].

Because the SMAS layer progressively thins out medially and disappears, biomechanical studies have found that there are differences in the viscoelasticity of the upper and lower regions of the SMAS [25]. It appears that biomechanically, the SMAS can be divided into two regions [25]:

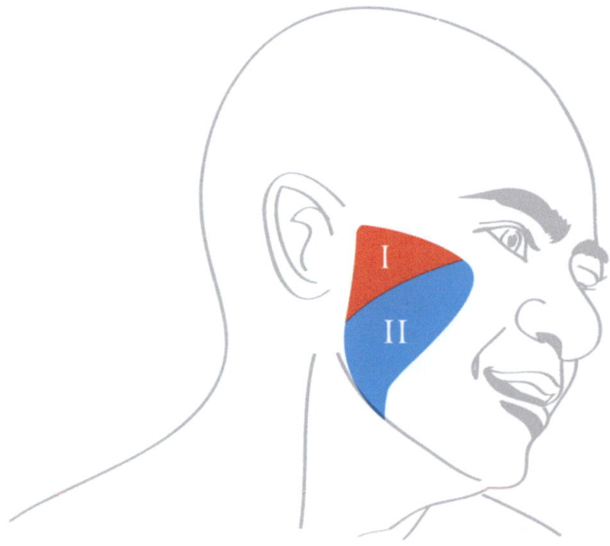

Fig. 11.1 SMAS zones of the face with the border between the zones making a natural subunit boundary

Region 1

Region 1 upper SMAS

This region is below the zygomatic arch, extending anterior of the tragus to the lateral edge of the zygomatic major muscle, then posteriorly to the upper edge of the platysma beneath the ear lobe. This triangular projection was denoted as the aponeurotic part of the pre-tragal SMAS, superficial to the parotid fascia.

Region 2 lower SMAS

This is the polygonal projection beneath region 1, superficial to the masseter fascia. It extends downward infero-laterally along the anterior edge of the masseter muscle, intersecting with the rim of the mandible.

Others have concluded that rather than viewing the SMAS as a single unit, as is the usual plastic surgical view, it is important to understand the distinct biomechanical differences that exist between the upper and lower regions of this layer [25]. The two different portions of the SMAS layer are illustrated in the figure (Fig. 11.1) and in this author's view form the anatomical boundary between the two cheek subunits—a line important from a biomechanical and aesthetic point of view.

11.3   The Subunits of the Cheek

We've just discussed skin lines and lines of maximum extensibility (LME), which are dependent on the orientation and stretching of the elastic fibres. However, while reconstructing the face after creating a defect it is important to match donor tissue to the recipient area as much as possible. Such cutaneous restoration of complete regions with a specific thickness was termed regional selective restoration, and the fragment of skin with the typical characteristic for a specific facial area was called a "regional aesthetic unit" by Gonzalez-Ulloa who first pioneered this method of facial reconstruction [26]. He summarized the advantages of regional unit principle of facial reconstruction or "selective regional restoration" by means of "aesthetic units" as follows: To conceal the borders of transplanted skin within the confines of the region in order to give each area the histological character and thickness that are specific to that region [26].

As this chapter focuses on biodynamic excisional skin tension (BEST) lines the focus will be on the cheek region where the SMAS layer gives the skin special tension considerations. The skin of the cheek can be divided into three regions—two regions on the cheek (essentially regions 1 and 2 described earlier) and a third infraorbital subunit where there is an increased risk of ectropion formation. As authors have noted, it may be occasionally necessary to sacrifice adjacent normal tissue, but final results are far superior when scars follow facial subunits, thus minimizing the risk of a patchwork-like appearance [27].

In areas like the nose, tissue is not very mobile and skin tension or BEST lines matter less than matching subunits with similar pilo-sebaceous skin. Nasal skin is unique when compared to non-nasal facial skin both in terms of dermal thickness and density of pilo-sebaceous units [28]. Rahman and others studied the histological aspects of regional units of the face and graded them both by thickness, and by the number of pilo-sebaceous units (Figs. 11.2 and 11.3).

Grade 1 <5 pilo-sebaceous units per 2.5 mm of skin
Grade II 6–10 pilo-sebaceous units per 2.5 mm of skin
Grade III >10 pilo-sebaceous units per 10 mm of skin

Other authors have sought to measure thickness of facial skin and corroborate previously described relative thickness indices [29]. The authors noted that the presence of abundant sebaceous glands results in a thicker dermis but this by itself does not interfere with the measurements of the epidermis or dermis, which are based on specific histological features [29]. Thickness of skin is also important because in reconstructive procedures, the goal is to replace like-with-like. The authors

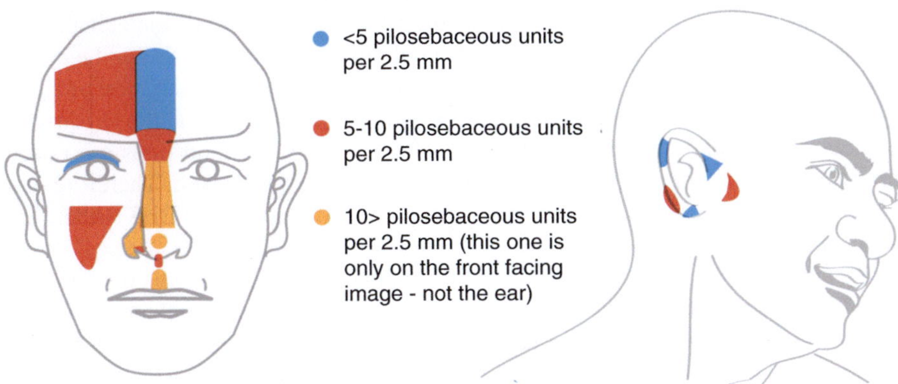

Fig. 11.2 Pilosebaceous units of the face

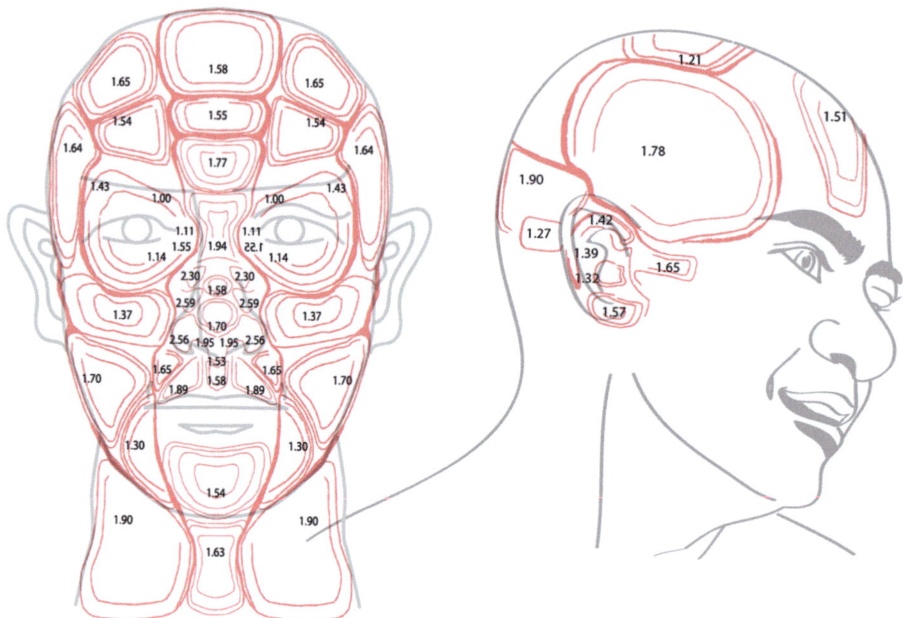

Fig. 11.3 Thickness of different regions of the face (in mm)

concluded that the area of the face with the thickest dermis was the lower nasal sidewall and the thinnest was the upper medial eyelid. The area with the thickest epidermis was the upper lip and the thinnest was the posterior auricular skin. Overall eyelid skin is the thinnest in the face. The thickest portions of the skin appeared to be in the lower nasal sidewall, but these were a good match for ala and post-auricular skin with implications when planning skin grafts. Interestingly, though there was no correlation between dermal and epidermal thickness, the former is more important in wound dynamics. As noted earlier, the thickest epidermis was found at the upper lip, and the thinnest epidermis was posterior auricular skin.

Thacker and others have emphasized the importance of skin biomechanics in plastic surgery, concluding that the direction of elliptical incisions should be correlated with the direction of reduced tension in the skin, resulting in narrower and less visible scars [30]. However, on the cheek only focusing on tension at the expense of neurovascular supply can be problematic—for example, if island flaps are raised from an area of lesser blood supply, whiteness of the flap may result. Therefore, not only does the skin closure need to consider skin tension and RSTL/BEST lines, but also neurovascular zones.

Bush calculated a median rotation of 30° in the long axis of wounds for different facial expressions. This was compared to a mean rotation of principal tension directions of 17° for wide opening of the mouth and 25° for smiling [31]. The rotation of the tension field during facial expressions may affect the appearance of a healed facial wound. The inclusion of *in vivo* tension in the face model is important [32]. Given biodynamic excision skin tension (BEST) line measurements include in vivo

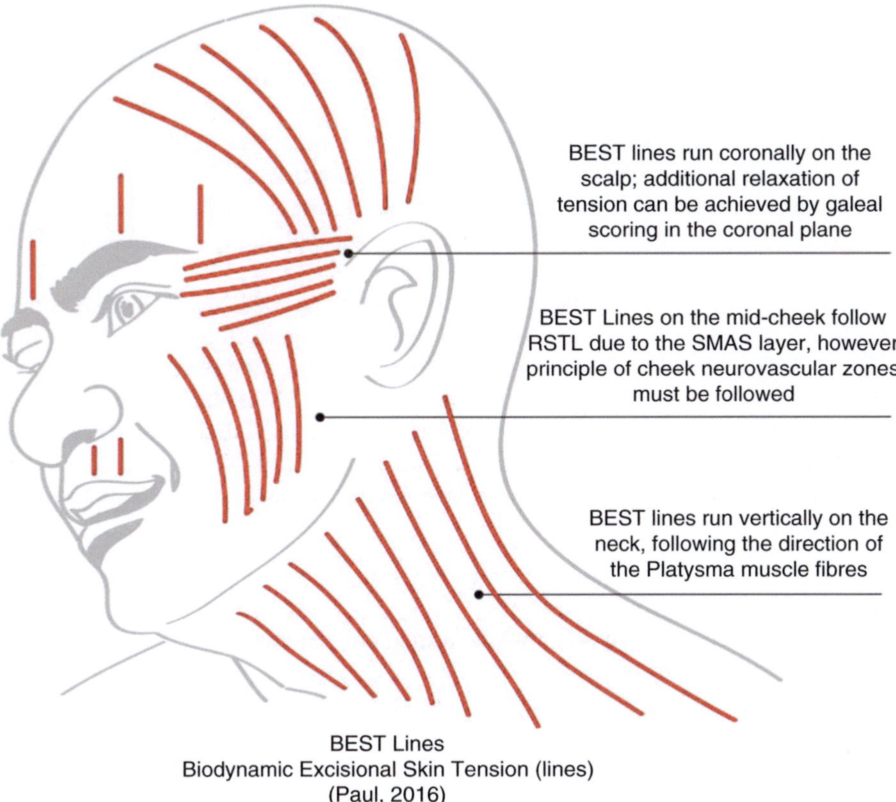

Fig. 11.4 Biodynamics Excisional Skin Tension (BEST) Lines variances from RSTL

assessments, they must be considered in addition to RSTL and the few variances are illustrated in Fig. 11.4.

11.4 Neurovascular Units of the Cheek

One of the interesting and yet underappreciated findings about skin tension is the effect on the underlying fat. Unlike the epidermis and dermis, the hypodermis or subcutaneous fat undergoes significant changes when the overlying skin is stretched. Adipocytes are compressed and diminished in size, leading to thinning of the subcutaneous layer [6]. In areas like the cheek, thinning out on one side will leave a noticeable mismatch, and therefore when closure entails significant wound tension, local flaps are often used. However, given the thinning of the subcutaneous tissue which may become apparent with age—often long after surgery, this author prefers to use island flaps as they thin out less due to the subcutaneous bulk provided by the island pedicle.

However, one of the dictums in plastic surgery is that flaps can pincushion; grafts do not. But over the mid-cheek, grafts give a less than optimal outcome due to colour and contour mismatch. Many island flaps can also appear whiter than surrounding skin post-operatively and therefore they have not been used as widely. If island flaps are planned with neurovascular zones in mind, they don't cause thinning of sub-cutis due to stretch (as any thinning of adipose tissue will not be noticeable) and can produce good results. In this section, neurovascular units of the cheek will be discussed with a case study to demonstrate the ideal planning of such flaps on the cheek, when primary closure is not possible.

Chandrawarkar and Cervino were first to delineate the cheek into five zones. While the rationale for their classification was to delineate the aesthetic subunits (Fig. 11.5) described by other authors [26], their classification described the neurovascular anatomy of the cheek [33]. This author has used a similar model in surgical practice. The anatomy of the cheek neurovascular subunits with respect to nerve and blood supply is illustrated here (Figs. 11.6 and 11.7).

The following are the cheek subunits (adapted from Chandrawarkar and Cervino's original description [32]:

Zone 1:
Superior: The lower eyelid crease
Lateral: Vertical line drawn downwards from lateral canthus
Inferior: Horizontal line from the nasal sill
Medial: Nasolabial crease and lateral margin of nose

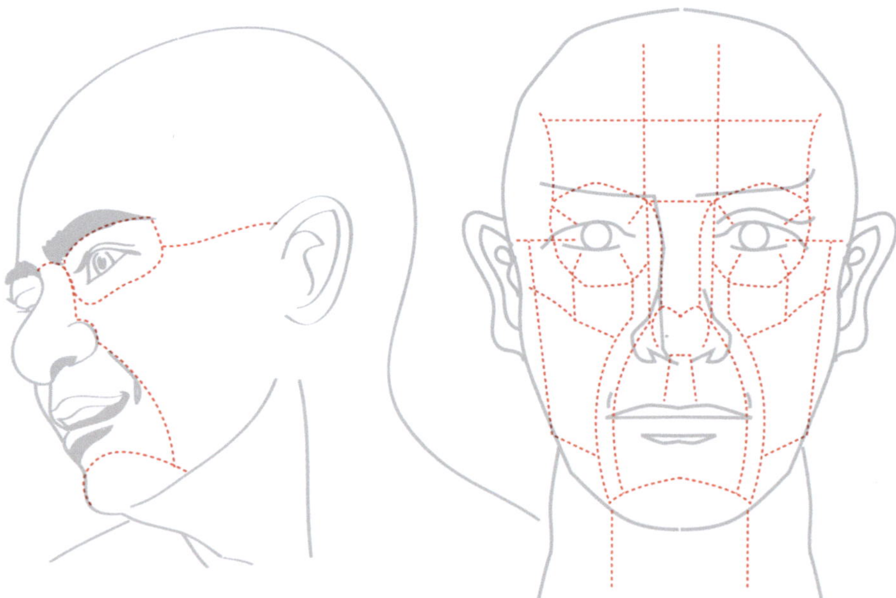

Fig. 11.5 Aesthetic subunits of the face

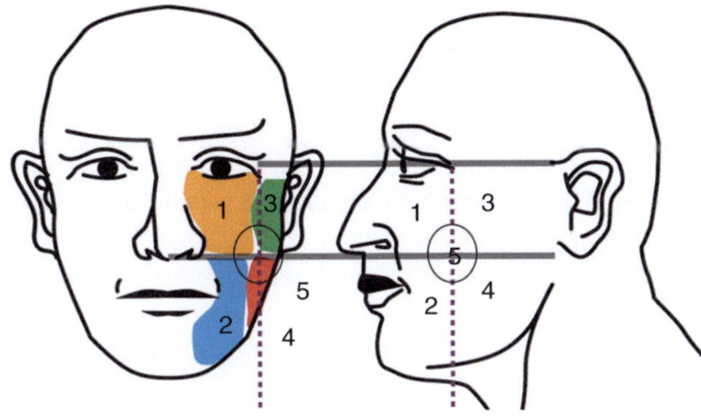

Fig. 11.6 Cheek neurovascular subunits

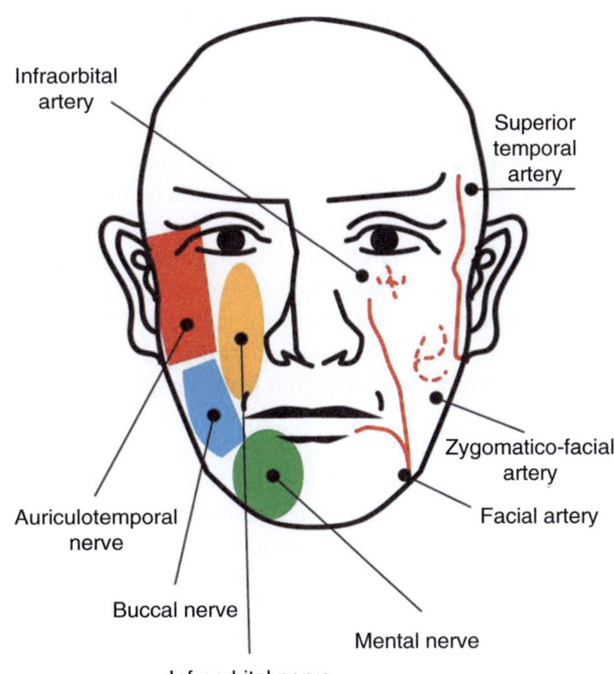

Fig. 11.7 Neurovascular anatomy of cheek

Zone 2:
Superior: Horizontal line from the nasal sill
Lateral: Vertical line from the lateral canthus
Inferior: The lower jawline
Medial: Vertical line from the angle of the mouth

Zone 3:
Superior: Horizontal line from the lateral canthus
Lateral: The pre-auricular crease

Inferior: Horizontal line from the nasal sill
Medial: Vertical line from lateral canthus

Zone 4:
Superior: Horizontal line from the nasal sill
Lateral: The pre-auricular crease and ascending ramus of mandible
Inferior: Lower jawline
Medial: Vertical line from the lateral canthus

Zone 5: Central circular zone, about 2 cm in diameter.

11.5   Surgical Algorithm for Reconstruction of Cheek Defects

Zone 1: Zone 1 defects are reconstructed bringing skin and subcutaneous tissue from zones 2 or 5. While some recommend V-Y advancement flaps [32], this author has found the oblique-sigmoid flap more useful in the mid-cheek due to its elliptical shape, allowing for a better contour when healed. In this author's view, the V-Y flap is more suitable for the naso-labial region rather than the mid cheek.

Zone 2: Zone 2 defects are reconstructed using any kind of a transposition flap below the jawline and the neck. The flaps can be tailored medially or laterally, taking into account the hair pattern of the beard area.

Zone 3: Zone 3 defects are reconstructed using a local transposition flap based medially. Here, hair distribution is the critical factor in determining the orientation of the flap.

Zone 4: Zone 4 defects usually need a medially-based transposition flap as there is better mobility in the medial direction.

Zone 5: Zone 5 defects usually are best reconstructed using rotational flaps from the angle of the jaw. And when mobilising skin from the neck region onto the cheek, the SMAS anatomy we have just discussed must be considered.

11.6   BEST Lines of the Face

A total of cases 418 were studied both pre-excision using the tensiometer previously described in detail [34]. Biodynamic excisional skin tension (BEST) lines of the face generally run along the RSTL (resting skin tension lines) (Fig. 11.8). However, there are some exceptions where BEST lines are more suitable (Fig. 11.4)—in the zygoma, the BEST lines run horizontally confining scarring to that subunit as well as preventing lateral pull on the eyelid; in the neck the BEST lines run vertically along the platysma muscle fibres. RSTL are illustrated in Fig. 11.8. Regions of the face where cleavage lines (Langer) and visual lines (wrinkle) contradict RSTL and BEST lines are illustrated in Figs. 11.9, 11.10, and 11.11.

Fig. 11.8 Relaxed skin tension lines (RSTL)

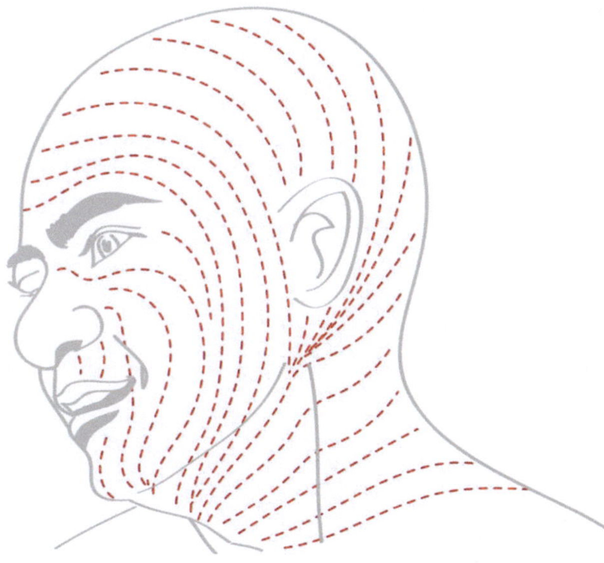

Fig. 11.9 Cleavage lines and where they contradict RSTL and BEST lines

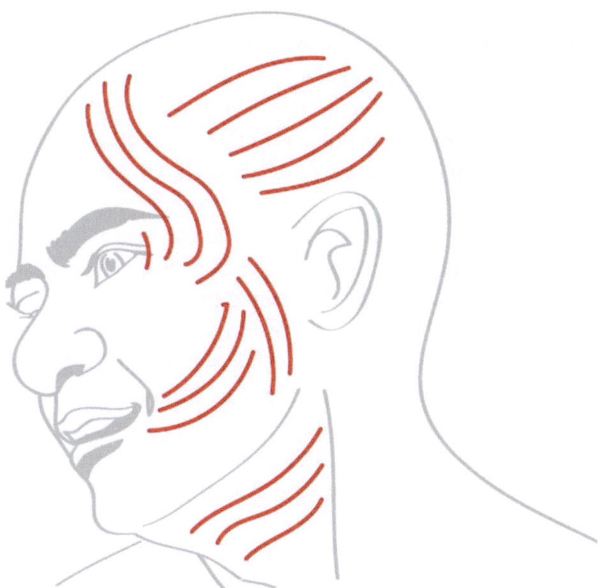

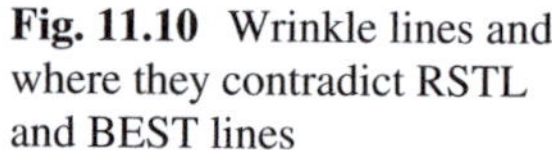

Fig. 11.10 Wrinkle lines and where they contradict RSTL and BEST lines

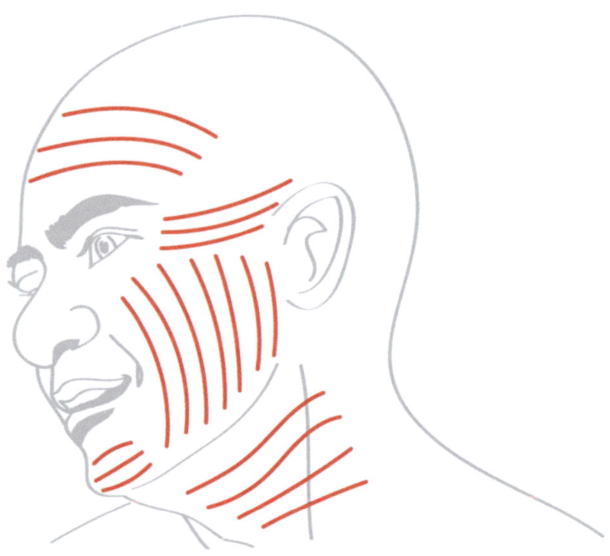

11.7   Case Study: Planning of Wound Closures Considering BEST Lines and Subunits

This patient (Fig. 11.12) presented with a lesion that was horizontally-orientated below the lower eyelid region. As we note from the BEST line illustration, closures under the eyelid need to be in the vertical direction to prevent ectropion formation—as an ectropion can occur well after the wound has healed. Given the width of the lesion, primary closure using BEST lines would create excessive tension and the resultant thinning of the hypodermis could lead to a mismatched appearance. In this case, the author planned an oblique-sigmoid island flap, the details of which have been the subject of a previous article [35]. This flap was chosen ahead of a V-Y advancement island flap (because the V-Y flap would have more lines of closure against BEST lines) or a rotation flap (as it would not be feasible from an optimal neurovascular zone). In this author's view, island flaps, when not planned from optimal neurovascular zones can lead to whiteness—and the end-result often resembles a skin graft. Others have noted that facial contour deformities affect the impression of an individual, with greater cognitive importance given to deformities of the central cheek [36] and therefore following BEST lines and neurovascular zones is important on the cheek.

As we can see from the images (Figs. 11.13 and 11.14), in this case-study, the flap is chosen from zone 5 because the defect lies in zone 1 (using the algorithm described earlier). The final closure causes no tension on the lower eyelid—and the primary-closure element of the flap also follows the BEST lines of the cheek. Choosing the optimal neurovascular zone means that the underlying blood

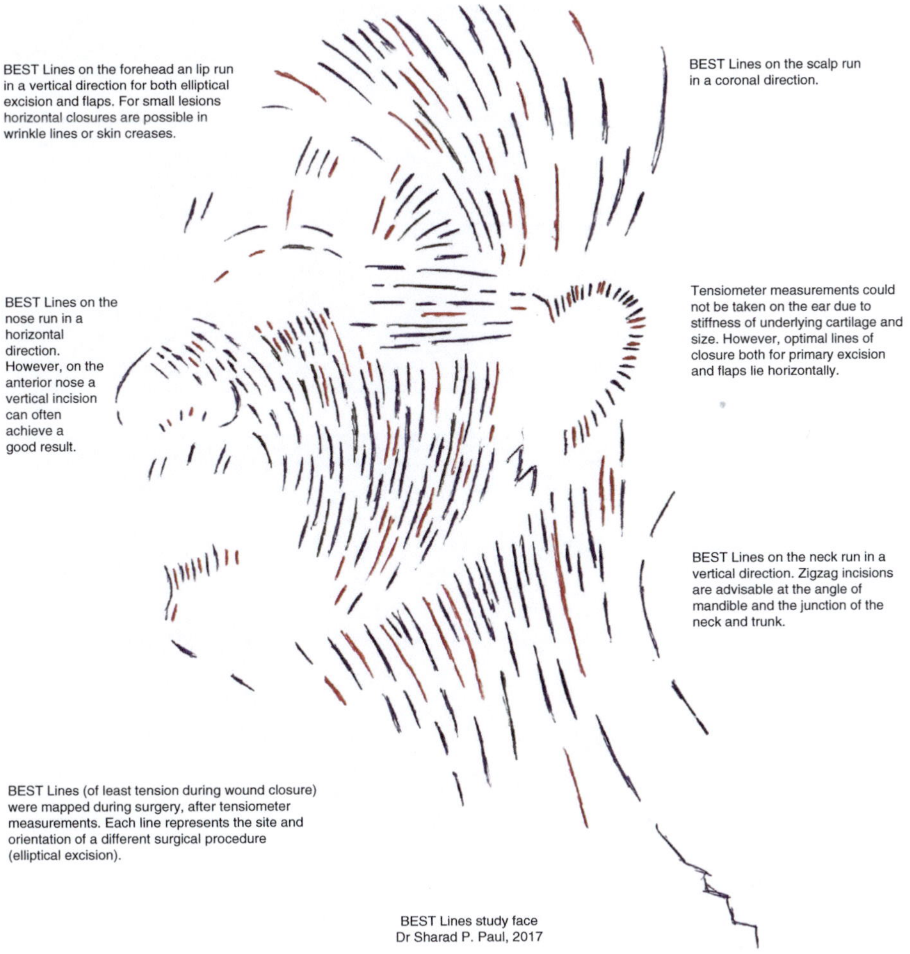

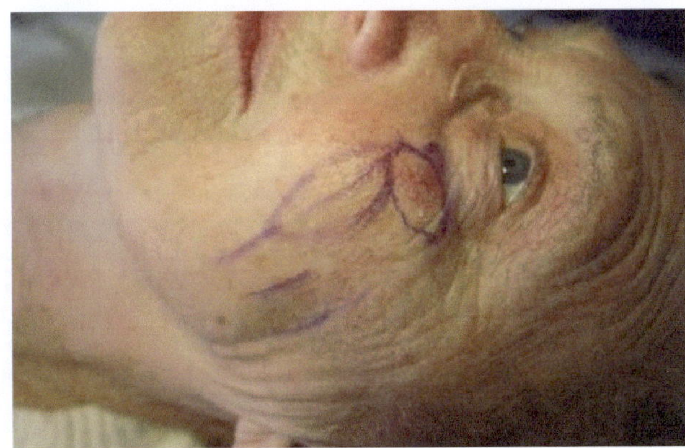

Fig. 11.11 BEST line study of head and neck lesions—each line represents the orientation of a different surgical excision. The clear preferential direction offers a good guide for cutaneous surgery of the face

Fig. 11.12 Lesion on the cheek located against BEST lines and therefore a flap is planned

Fig. 11.13 The flap is raised from zone 5. Island flap is chosen to reduce any contour defect due to thinning of fat, and from the optimal neurovascular zone to avoid whiteness of the flap post-operatively

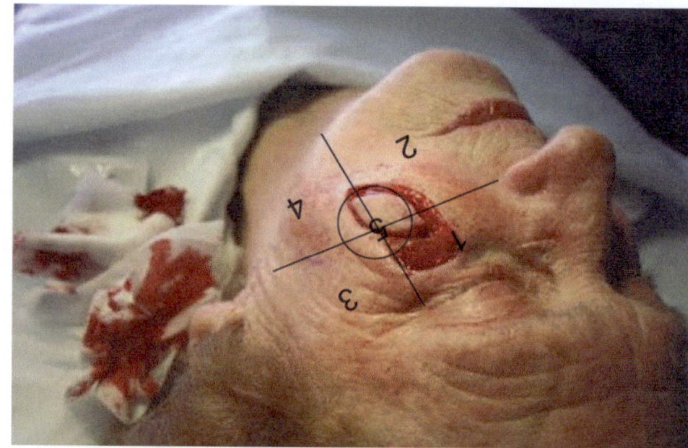

Fig. 11.14 Oblique-sigmoid island flap sutured in place with no contour defect or tension on eyelid and closure along BEST lines

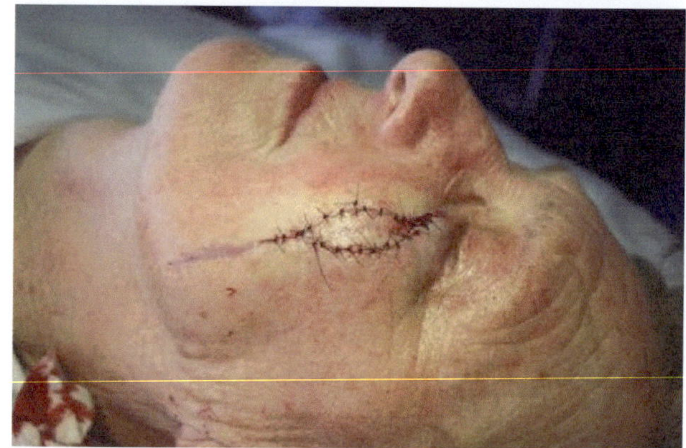

supply is similar between donor and recipient areas—and therefore does not cause any post-operative whiteness or suffusion of the area. We can now see how BEST lines still determine wound closures—as the reduced tension that results causes less scarring, and also avoids thinning of underlying fat. However on the face, for optimal colour-matching, one also needs to consider neurovascular zones.

References

1. Menick FJ. Defects of the nose, lip, and cheek: rebuilding the composite defect. Plast Reconstr Surg. 2007;120:887–98.
2. Dunlavey E, Leshin B. The simple excision. Dermatol Clin. 1998;16:49–64.
3. Goldberg LH. Cold steel surgery: the ellipse. In: Lask GP, Moy RL, editors. Principles and techniques of cutaneous surgery. New York: McGraw-Hill; 1996. p. 165–70.
4. Paul SP. Skin, a biography. 4th Estate. New York: HarperCollins; 2013. p. 182.
5. Baker SR. Fundamentals of expanded tissue. Head Neck. 1991;13:327–33.
6. Zöllner AM, Holland MA, Honda KS, Gosain AK, Kuhl E. Growth on demand: reviewing the mechanobiology of stretched skin. J Mech Behav Biomed Mater. 2013;2013(28):495–509.

7. McGrath JA, Uitto J. Chapter 3: Anatomy and organization of human skin. In: Burns T, Breathnach S, Cox N, Griffiths C, editors. Rook's textbook of dermatology, vol. 1. 8th ed. Oxford: Blackwell; 2010.

8. De Filippo RE, Atala A. Stretch and growth: the molecular and physiologic influences of tissue expansion. Plast Reconstr Surg. 2002;109:2450–62.

9. Austad ED, Pasy KA, McClatchey KD, Cheery GW. Histomorphologic evaluation of guinea pig skin and soft tissue after controlled tissue expansion. Plast Reconstr Surg. 1982;70:704–10.

10. Karl Langer. Zur Anatomie und Physiologie der Haut. Über die Spaltbarkeit der Cutis. Sitzungsbericht der Mathematisch-naturwissenschaftlichen Classe der Wiener Kaiserlichen Academie der Wissenschaften 1861; Abt 44.

11. Kocher E. Chirurgische Operationslekre, Jena; 1892.

12. Maranda EL, Heifetz R, Cortizo J, Hafeez F, Nouri K. Kraissl lines—a map. JAMA Dermatol. 2016;152(9):1014.

13. Cox HT. The cleavage lines of the skin. Br J Surg. 1941;29(114):234–40.

14. Kraissl CJ. The selection of appropriate lines for elective surgical incisions. Plast Reconstr Surg. 1951;8(1):1–28.

15. Kraissl CJ, Conway H. Excision of small tumours of the skin of the face with special reference to the wrinkle lines. Surgery. 1949;25:592.

16. Rubin LR. Langer's lines and facial scars. Plast Reconstr Surg. 1948;3:147.

17. Borges AF. Relaxed skin tension lines (RSTL) versus other skin lines. Plast Reconstr Surg. 1984;73(1):144–50.

18. McGrath JA, Eady RA, Pope FM. Rook's textbook of dermatology. 7th ed. Oxford: Blackwell; 2004. p. 31.

19. Mitz V, Peyronie M. The superficial musculo aponeurotic system (SMAS) in the parotid and cheek area. Plast Reconstr Surg. 1976;58(1):80–8.

20. Macchi V, Tiengo C, Porzionato A, et al. Histotopographic study of the fibroadipose connective cheek system. Cells Tissues Organs. 2009;191(1):47–56.

21. Broughton M, Fyfe GM. The superficial musculoaponeurotic system of the face: a model explored. Anat Res Int. 2013;2013:794682.

22. Khawaja HA, et al. SMAFS (Superficial Musculoaponeurotic-Fatty System): a changed SMAS concept; anatomic variants, modes of handling, and clinical significance in facelift surgery. Advanced surgical facial rejuvenation. New York: Springer; 2011. p. 35–45.

23. Har-Shai Y, et al. Viscoelastic properties of the Superficial Musculoaponeurotic System (SMAS): a microscopic and mechanical study. Aesthet Plast Surg. 1997;21:219–24.

24. Hirshowitz B, Jackson IT. An attempt to harness the viscoelastic properties of skin in face lift operations. A preliminary report. Ann Plast Surg. 1987;18:188–98.

25. Hu X, Wang Z, Wang Q, Zhang C, Hu G, Qin H. Are there differences between the upper and lower parts of the superficial musculoaponeurotic system? A preliminary biomechanical study. Aesthet Surg J. 2014;34(5):661–7.

26. Gonzalez-Ulloa M. Restoration of the face covering by means of selected skin in regional aesthetic units. Br J Plast Surg. 1956;9(3):212–21.

27. Cordeiro PG, Santamaria E. Free flap reconstruction of the cheek. Oper Tech Plast Reconstr Surg. 1999;6(4):265–74.

28. Rahman M, Jefferson N, Stewart DA. The histology of facial aesthetic subunits: implications for common nasal reconstructive procedures. J Plast Reconstr Aesthet Surg. 2010;63(5):753–6.

29. Chopra K, Calva D, et al. A comprehensive examination of topographic thickness of skin in the human face. Aesthet Surg J. 2015;35(8):1007–13.

30. Thacker JG, Stalnecker MC, Allaire PE, Edgerton MT, Rodeheaver GT, Edlich RF. Practical applications of skin biomechanics. Clin Plast Surg. 1977;4(2):167–71.

31. Bush J, Ferguson MWJ, Mason T, McGrouther G. The dynamic rotation of Langer's lines on facial expression. J Plast Reconstr Aesthet Surg. 2007;60(4):393–9.

32. Flynn C, Stavness I, Lloyd J, Fels S. A finite element model of the face including an orthotropic skin model under in vivo tension. Comput Methods Biomech Biomed Engin. 2015;18(6):571–82.

33. Chandawarkar RY, Cervino AL. Subunits of the cheek: an algorithm for the reconstruction of partial-thickness defects. Br J Plast Surg. 2003;56(2):135–9.
34. Paul SP, et al. A new skin tensiometer device: computational analyses to understand biodynamic excisional skin tension lines. Sci Rep. 2016;6:30117.
35. Paul SP. Islands on the cheek: island flaps on the cheek and a modified oblique-sigmoid flap. In: Paul SP, Norman RA, editors. Clinical cases in skin cancer surgery and treatment. Geneva: Springer; 2016. p. 21–31.
36. Rankin M, Borah GL. Perceived functional impact of abnormal facial appearance. Plast Reconstr Surg. 2003;111:72140–6.

Chapter 12
Patterns, Biomechanics and Behaviour

It has been noted in scientific literature that humans are the only mammal to have whorl patterns on the scalp, and that each human has a unique pattern [1]. While a literature review does not prove any contrary view, this matched this author's observations on apes, where scalp whorls seem conspicuous by their absence. The author is also an animal biologist and often asked to operate or examine animals, especially apes with skin tumours or dermatological conditions (Fig. 12.1).

One of the major methods to understand the nature vs. nurture aspect of any aetiology is to undertake twin studies, as monozygotic twins are 100% genetically similar, whereas dizygotic twins are on average only 50% similar for segregating genes—and such twin studies help us untangle genetic and environmental influences [2]. There was a report on monozygotic twins (dichorionic monozygotic twin boys), that showed that one twin had a single hair whorl—opening in a clockwise direction, while the second twin had two hair whorls—each opening in opposite directions [3]. Wunderlich and Heerema had previously suggested hair whorl patterns are established in utero, and therefore evident at birth [1]. How much of this hair patterning is genetic and what are the possible mechanical causes? This article reviews the types of hair whorl patterns, the mechanisms behind the development of scalp whorls and their surgical implications.

© Springer International Publishing AG, part of Springer Nature 2018

S. P. Paul, *Biodynamic Excisional Skin Tension Lines for Cutaneous Surgery*,

https://doi.org/10.1007/978-3-319-71495-0_12

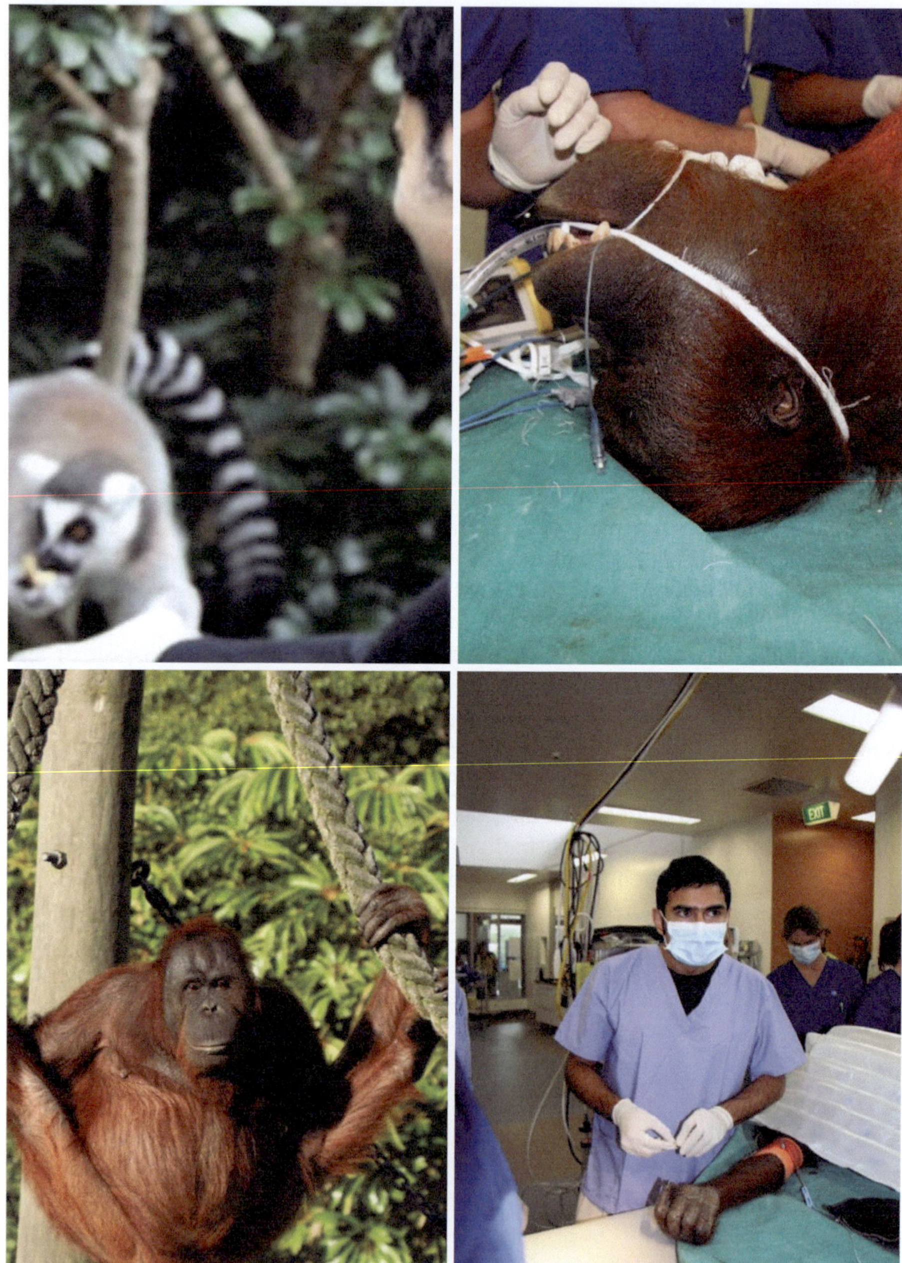

Fig. 12.1 Author's work as an animal biologist did not reveal whorl patterns on scalps of apes

12.1   Developmental Theories and Hair Patterns

While hair on the scalp of primates may seem plentiful compared to humans, humans have more hair follicles per unit area than higher primates [4]. A study of hair follicle patterns in foetal life is also useful, because the sequence of events that result in hair follicle patterns in foetal life is partially recapitulated in each cycle of follicular activity [5]. It must be also noted that all scalp hairs, except those of the occipital region, are in the same growth phase until about 7 months after birth [5]. While all hair follicles grow obliquely in relation to the epidermis, it is only at the parietal scalp that we see the classical whorl pattern that usually assumes the golden spiral pattern. Contrary to twin studies on scalp whorls that showed differences between twins, Kiil's Norwegian study of frontal hair patterns (not whorls) showed a complete concordance between uni-ovular twins, suggesting that the formation of scalp whorls is not predominantly genetic or inherited [6]. In his study, Kiil described three hair patterns, Type I (downwards), Type II (upwards and downwards) and Type III (upwards)—and later noted the preponderance of Type III patterns in those diagnosed with Down's Syndrome [7].

The hair whorl becomes visible on the "crown" of the human head between the 10th and the 18th week of gestation [8]. This period is characterized by extraordinarily rapid growth of the brain secondary to the major wave of neuroblast replication, and therefore theories abound regarding the formation of scalp whorls and morphogenesis of the hair follicles of the scalp [9]. Studies suggest that especially on the scalp, expansion and tension are interrelated i.e. when skin is expanded or stretched, the deformation gradient has an elastic and a growth part [10]. These activities all seem to respond to changes in surface tension. Some authors therefore attribute a key role for surface tension in such tightly controlled processes of development such as epithelial morphogenesis [11]. The finite element theory of skin tension has many molecular mechanisms, including factors like intermediate filaments, microfilaments, and microtubules—as well as extracellular elements such as collagen, elastin and glycosaminoglycan [8]. Contours of skin tension have been studied by many pioneers such as Langer, who mapped skin tension lines using a round-tipped awl to create defects in cadaveric skin, and then observing the elongation of these circular defects due to the underlying wound tension [11]. Jacquet and others noted that skin behaves differently *in vivo* and *ex vivo*—for example, if one observed the shape of the *ex vivo* test, the stress-strain curve starts with a very low slope and then presents a large non-linearity at low strain, whereas in an *in vivo* test, the curve is much stiffer [12].

One thing we know is that hair patterns on the scalp are no different to hair patterns on areas of the body such as the limbs i.e. the downgrowth of follicles is not vertical but oblique [8]. This fact, when considered along with the stiffness of skin during the initial stress phase of skin, gave rise to several mechanical theories on the development of scalp whorl patterns. But is this due to intrauterine or gestational factors, and is this genetically pre-determined?

Behavioural studies in ungulate animals like cattle seem to have a common theme: subjects with higher facial whorls are significantly more 'reactive' than those with lower facial whorls and more suspicious of strangers [13]. With ponies, those with whorls positioned to the left tend to be more affable in their behaviour when compared to ponies with whorls on the right [14]. Therefore, for those in the business of buying horses, hair whorls have become a method of selection—with ponies with right-sided whorls scoring higher for wariness, associated flightiness and unfriendliness, and therefore ending up less desirable [14]. The horse is no longer evolving by Natural Selection—rather, the *Equus* species has become subject to Artificial Selection, dictating which individuals are bred as part of strict breeding programmes, with the aim of modulating equine temperaments [13], Therefore horses end up with limited scalp whorl patterns [13]. Ponies with multiple i.e. three facial whorls are found to exhibit greater wariness than those horses with one single facial whorl; ponies rated as the most enthusiastic typically had two facial whorls. Facial hair whorls among animals may provide a physical feature which could be used to make a rapid assessment of temperament, as we discussed earlier.

These animal studies led researchers to look at multiple scalp whorl patterns in humans as indicators of behaviour. A study published of hair whorl pattern in schizophrenics [14] was interesting as it found that the frequency distribution of hair whorl patterns for those with a single hair whorl was significantly different between the schizophrenic and normal subjects ($p = 0.01$) [15]. However, when multiple whorls were studied, the frequency distribution of bilateral, left, midline, and right hair whorls in schizophrenic subjects was not significantly different than normal ($p = 0.80$) [15]. This study, by Alexander's team [15], compared the orientation of single hair whorls in 49 schizophrenic patients with those from four independent studies. This aroused considerable interest and led to others attempting to replicate this study [16]. A study undertaken of *parietal* scalp whorl *patterns* (not *frontal* hair *direction*) in schizophrenics revealed that patients with anticlockwise hair whorls were not found to have any factor in common, other than a diagnosis of schizophrenia [16].

Other studies looked at brain hemispheric differences to see if this would add anything to this discussion. We know that the left hemisphere tends to be the dominant hemisphere for language and manual dexterity, and therefore people looked at right- or left-handedness and scalp whorls. Effectively, any positive association would prove a link between a *structural lateralization* marker (hair-whorl direction) and the *functional lateralization* markers (handedness) [17]. Klar proposed a genetic model based on a single random-recessive gene with two alleles that control both handedness and hair-whorl orientation [18]. To investigate this theory further, a large study was undertaken wherein 1212 individuals were investigated for handedness and scalp hair-whorl direction [17]. The team additionally studied hemispheric language dominance by using functional transcranial Doppler sonography (fTCD), because this method's ability to measure cerebral perfusion changes during neural activation makes is extremely useful in neuroimaging [17]. This study could not find the expected association between hair-whorl direction and either language dominance or handedness.

How many whorls can a person have? A recent study was published about a 5-year old boy who presented with six whorls—four clockwise and two anticlockwise. This led to a flurry of interest in the child's neurological and cranial development. But as the researchers noted, "He was born from a non-consanguineous marriage with an uneventful antepartum period. His physical and mental development were as expected for age. The family history was unremarkable, and none of his family members had abnormal scalp whorl patterns. His dermatoglyphics were normal and he was right-handed. Magnetic resonance imaging of the brain and blood karyotyping were normal [19]." This revealed the possibility that "abnormal" hair patterns could indeed occur with a normal phenotype.

Perhaps the better way to look at the scalp whorls is considering that it is the gestational period that matters i.e. the 10–17th week is the key period for the determination of both hair whorl patterns and foetal brain development [20] and this has led researchers in the search for mechanical theories of scalp whorl formation.

12.2   Mechanical Theories

D'Arcy Thompson wrote in *Growth and Form* [21]: "Among the forces which determine the forms of cells, whether they be solitary or arranged in contact with one another, this force of surface-tension is certainly of great, and paramount importance." Ludwig [22] was possibly the first person to correlate this surface-tension specifically with hair follicle streams with growth patterns and look for investigate associations between the different whorl shapes. Ludwig classified growth "disturbances" into divergent whorls, convergent whorls, and crosses [22].

Surface tension must be viewed alongside skin tension, as the latter is important in planning wound closures, with the aim being to reduce skin tension. Skin tension can be considered morphogenetic and ends up directing the formation of data acquisition structures such as hair follicles [23]. Computational analysis of the skin tension fields must therefore be considered under the finite element theory, with an emphasis on molecular and supramolecular structures within skin that resist the deformation gradient [24]. Others have used computational methods to measure skin tension to help understand skin lines of tension and the cleavage planes of skin [25].

Epidermal Growth Factor (EGF), a single chained polypeptide, is neither a nutrient nor a structural protein, but is a potent hormonal stimulator of cell division. EGF acts by binding to specific receptor macromolecules located within the cellular plasma membrane [26]. Crucially EGF plays a major part in hair follicle and craniofacial development, and the administration of EGF in mice causes angular deflections of hair follicles in a single plane, like the slanting that occurs in scalp whorls [27]. Eyelid un-fusion, a major developmental occurrence in the craniofacial region, is a relatively small alteration in cell surface binding, that ends up causing a very large variation in systemic organization of the body. EGF also plays a major role in eyelid un-fusion, and authors have noted that such controlled processes that require a great degree of amplification are more prone to developmental pattern variations [28]. Hoath believed that rather than acceleration, what happened during such regulated processes is that the EGF alters the surface tension of the organism [29].

Given it is now known that EGF plays a major role in hair follicle sloping and whorl formation, does it also influence the actual geometric spiral pattern? In vitro studies have shown that EGF indeed affects tissue organization and pattern formation—and studies on populations of human keratinocytes reveal that, under the influence of EGF, the formation of whorls and ridges occur [30]. We have just discussed that EGF helps the formation of whorls, and other authors have noted that in the early period of wound healing, factors such as transforming growth factor (TGF)-β, platelet-derived growth factor (PDGF), and epidermal growth factor (EGF) are extensively involved [31]; EGF especially may reduce scar formation or minimise contour deformity during the healing process [31]. However, the golden spiral pattern noted in scalp whorls is unique for a variety of reasons—the association of this pattern to the developing human brain enlargement (neocortex), the absence of this pattern's existence in other advanced primates, and the fact that this scalp whorl pattern is related to mathematically well-studied growth curves such as the logarithmic spiral has led to studies on the specific biomechanics of the spiral pattern [21]. After Langer's pioneering work on skin cleavage lines, many others have noted the relationship between Langer's Lines and hair follicles—and experimental studies have shown that there is a good correlation between Langer's Lines and direction of hair streams [32].

12.3   The Golden Spiral and Surgical Applications

Ludwig's assumed that scalp whorls represented a topological sphere where an irreducible minimum of two whorls represented the basic disturbances occurring during development [22]. He mooted that the sum of the divergent and convergent whorls -2 would equal the number of crosses found [22]. His observations were indeed not dissimilar to Euler's famous mathematical identity $e^{i\pi} + 1 = 0$ [33]. Euler introduced into the equation the concept of infinity, and the pattern became an endless logarithmic circle around the origin, the golden spiral [33].

Recently an experiment was conducted using saline expanders to study if pressure can create enough shearing forces to replicate the dermo-epidermal shear that occurs during scalp whorl formation, and thereby replicate the slanting of hair follicles [34]. The purpose of this experiment was to prove the mechanical theory of scalp whorl formation i.e. to see if the causation of shearing forces between the uppermost two layers of pigskin (the epidermis and fatty dermis) would result in the formation of spirals along an advancing front [34]. The study, by this author, concluded that, under certain conditions, rapid tissue expansion can cause dermoepidermal shear, which in turn can result in the formation of spiral patterns such as the golden spiral along an expanding front [34].

The mechanical theory of scalp whorl formation has important surgical applications. Noting the effect of EGF on the formation of scalp whorls, other studies have noted that EGF mediates wound contractility through the stimulation of myofibroblast proliferation and therefore EGF reduces scar width or area not only through rapid epithelization, but also by contracting the wound [35]. This opens up avenues for further research into wound healing and scar reduction. The scalp donor area is a major factor in planning hair transplant surgery, and authors have shown that predicting the permanent safe donor area for hair transplantation in people with male pattern baldness can be done using the location of the parietal scalp whorl as an indicator [36]. Given experimental studies have shown the golden spiral pattern to be a pattern of rapid expansion [34], the golden spiral pattern has served as a useful surgical template when planning cutaneous flaps [37]. A study by this author confirmed that when a flap was planned using the golden spiral pattern, it allowed a surgeon to close the wound under less tension, when compared to standard rotational flaps. The mean reduction in tension, using the golden spiral pattern flap was estimated at around 25% [37].

Numerous studies have confirmed that skin wounds which are under mechanical tension are more prone to heal with the formation of a scar, and this led to current practice where surgeons aim to reduce tension at incision sites post-surgery [38] and that was the rationale behind this author's inquisition into BEST lines that led to this book. However, the fact that the skin's tensile stress has such a profound effect on wound healing indicates that there is a cellular mechanism at the wound-site by which stress is sensed and transduced to a physiological response. Most evidence points to cells in the connective tissue of the wound bed—fibroblasts or their relations, the myofibroblasts—as mediators of this mechanism [39]. Myofibroblasts have been known to draw wound edges together. Many animal models have demonstrated that changes in tension promote the proliferation of these cells, inhibits their apoptosis and activates many signalling pathways that may modify the deposition of ECM [40]. Cellular signalling by soluble molecules, such as growth factors are involved with physical patterning in animals. Threshold concentrations of signalling molecules have been known for many years to regulate the positioning and patterning of an organism's tissues—and these reaction-diffusion mechanisms, originally proposed by Turing [41], have been noted to be responsible for hair patterning in animals [42]. Until now we have been discussing mainly wound tension and biomechanics. Increasingly there is evidence to suggest that cells do not just passively respond to force—they actively respond to their environment by exerting force on it themselves and then responding to this "feel" [39].

12.4   Conclusion

Scalp whorls are more than a human curiosity—they are the pattern for mechanical expansion when the neocortex develops, and such deformation of hair follicles and arrangement into the logarithmic spiral pattern (Fig. 12.2) is modulated by proteins

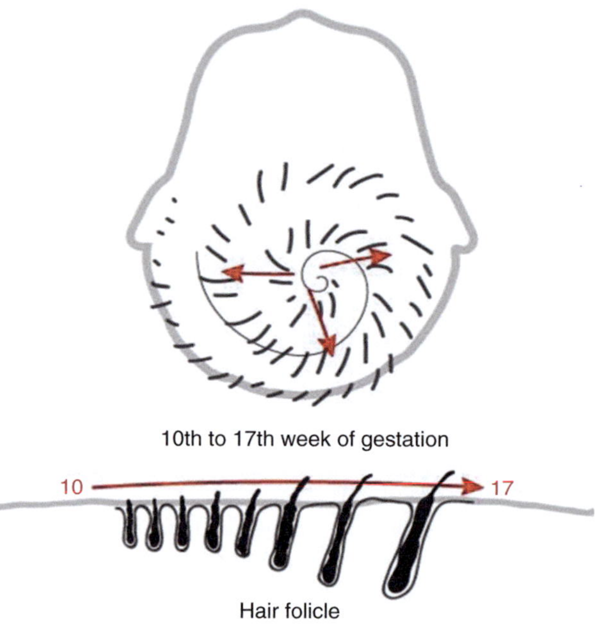

Fig. 12.2 Illustration of the deformation of hair follicles and arrangement of whorls into the logarithmic spiral pattern that occurs with rapid expansion of the neocortex

such as (but not limited to) the epidermal growth factor (EGF). The golden spiral pattern that occurs in scalp whorls, that has been discussed earlier, is merely a pattern of rapid expansion [34]. However, while scalp whorl patterns are different between individuals, they show no association with handedness or twinning. However, people suffering from schizophrenia have been noted to have abnormal scalp whorl patterns. Does this indicate maternal factors during weeks 10–17 of pregnancy play a part? All these areas are avenues for further research. In medicine, as specialties have become increasingly divided into silos there is a tendency to separate the biomechanics (physical) from behaviour (mental). This study into scalp whorl formation and patterns suggests that such an approach is scientifically unwise. A lecture based on these conclusions was presented by this author in a recent lecture at the Mayo Auditorium [43].

In conclusion, I would like to quote Aristotle, who wisely noted that skin was our *only* essential sense organ—necessary for being, and not just well-being— for without touch, there can be no life. Aristotle wrote: "In all disciplines in which there is systematic knowledge of things with principles, causes, or elements, it arises from a grasp of those: we think we have knowledge of a thing when we have found its primary causes and principles, and followed it back to its elements. Clearly, then, systematic knowledge of nature must start with an attempt to settle questions about principles" [44]. And that was what this book set out to do with respect to skin lines—understand their biology, biomechanics and behaviour.

Joint Grand Rounds Lecture

SURGERY, BIOMECHANICS AND BEHAVIOR & A WRITER'S GUIDE TO SURGICAL DIAGNOSIS

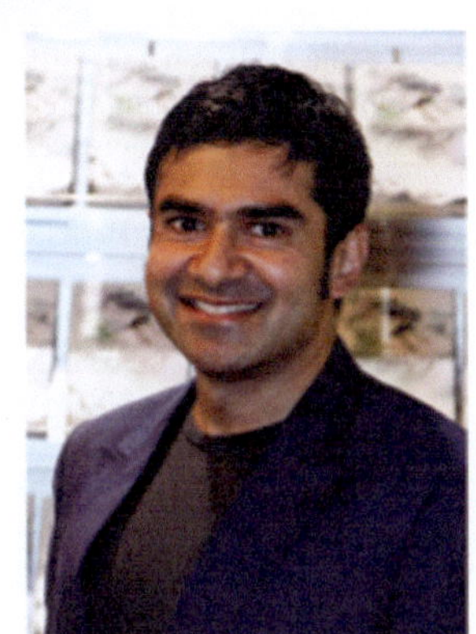

Sharad Paul, MD

Adjunct Professor, Auckland University of Technology, New Zealand
Senior Lecturer in Surgery and Skin Cancer, Universities of Auckland and Queensland

Tuesday, April 11, 2017

Grand Rounds
7:00 A.M.
Mayo Auditorium

UNIVERSITY OF MINNESOTA

References

1. Wunderlich RC, Heerema NA. Hair crown patterns of human newborns. Studies on parietal hair whorl locations and their directions. Clin Pediatr. 1975;14:1045–9. https://doi.org/10.1177/000992287501401111.
2. Bell JT, Saffery R. The value of twins in epigenetic epidemiology. Int J Epidemiol. 2012;41(1):140–50. https://doi.org/10.1093/ije/dyr179.
3. Hair whorls and monozygosity. J Invest Dermatol. 2004;122(4):1057–58. doi:https://doi.org/10.1111/j.0022–202X.2004.22420.x.
4. Goodhart CB. The evolutionary significance of human hair patterns and skin colouring. Adv Sci. 1960;17:53–8.
5. Dawber RPR. The embryology and development of human scalp hair. Clin Dermatol. 1988;6(4):1–6. https://doi.org/10.1016/0738–081X(88)90059–4.
6. Kiil V. Inheritance of frontal hair direction in man. J Hered. 1948;39:206–9.
7. Kiil V. Frontal hair direction in mentally deficient individuals. J Hered. 1948;39:281–5.
8. Hoath SB. Considerations on the role of surface tension and epidermal growth factor in the mechanism of integumental pattern formation. J Theor Biol. 1990;143:1–14.

9. Smith DW. Morphogenesis and malformation of the face and brain, Birth defects: original article series, vol. 11. New York: Alan R. Liss; 1975. p. 7.
10. Garikipati K. The kinematics of biological growth. Appl Mech Rev. 2009;62(3):030801.
11. Langer K. On the anatomy and physiology of the skin (1861), The Imperial Academy of Science, Vienna. Br J Plast Surg. 1978;17(31):93–106.
12. Jacquet E, Josse G, et al. A new experimental method for measuring skin's natural tension. Skin Res Technol. 2008;14:1–7.
13. Randle HD. Facial hair whorl position and temperament in cattle. Appl Anim Behav Sci. 1998;56:139–47.
14. Randle H, Webb TG, Gill LJ. The relationship between facial hair whorls and temperament in Lundy ponies. Annual report of the Lundy Field. Society. 2003;52:67–83.
15. Alexander RC. Increased incidence of counter-clockwise scalp hair whorl orientation in Caucasian schizophrenic patient. J Schizophr Res. 1993;9(2):145–6.
16. Puri BK, et al. Parietal scalp hair whorl patterns in schizophrenia. Biol Psychiatry. 1995;37(4):278–9.
17. Jansen A, Lohmann H, et al. The association between scalp hair-whorl direction, handedness and hemispheric language dominance: is there a common genetic basis of lateralization? Neuroimage Clin. 2007;35(2):853–61. https://doi.org/10.1016/j.neuroimage.2006.12.025.
18. Klar AJS. Human handedness and scalp hair-whorl direction develop from a common genetic mechanism. Genetics. 2003;165:269–76.
19. Malathi M. Multiple hair whorls in a child with normal cranial and neurologic development. Pediatr Dermatol. 2013;30(5):630–1.
20. Grandin T. Behavioural principles of livestock handling. Prof Anim Sci. 1989;5:1–11.
21. Thompson DW. On growth and form. New York: Cambridge University Press/Macmillan; 1945. p. 351.
22. Ludwig E. Morphologie und Morphogenehe des Haarstrichs. Z Anat Entwicklungsgeschaht. 1921;62(1):59–152.
23. Smith DW, Gong BT. Scalp-hair patterning: its origin and significance relative to early brain and upper facial development. Teratology. 1974;9:17–34.
24. Gordon R. A review of the theories of vertebrate neurulation and their relationship to the mechanics of neural tube birth defects. J Embryol Exp Morphol. 1985;89(Suppl):229–55.
25. Paul SP, et al. A new skin tensiometer device: computational analyses to understand biodynamic excisional skin tension lines. Sci Rep. 2016;6:30117. https://doi.org/10.1038/srep30117.
26. Carpenter G, Cohen S. Epidermal growth factor. Annu Rev Biochem. 1979;48:193–216.
27. Moore GP, et al. Effects of epidermal growth factor on hair growth in the mouse. J Endocrinol. 1981;88:293–9.
28. Thom R. Structural stability and morphogenesis. Reading: W. A. Benjamin; 1975.
29. Hoath SB. Considerations on the role of surface tension and epidermal growth factor in the mechanism of integumental pattern formation. J Theor Biol. 1990;143:9.
30. Green H, Thomas J. Pattern formation by cultured human epidermal cells: development of curved ridges resembling dermatoglyphs. Science. 1978;200:1385–8.
31. Kim YS, Lew DH, Tark KC, Rah DK, Hong JP. Effect of recombinant human epidermal growth factor against cutaneous scar formation in murine full-thickness wound healing. J Korean Med Sci. 2010;25(4):589–96.
32. Kwak M, Son D, Kim J, Han K. Static Langer's line and wound contraction rates according to anatomical regions in a porcine model. Wound Repair Regen. 2014;22(5):678–82. https://doi.org/10.1111/wrr.12206.
33. Simmons L. The baffling and beautiful wormhole between branches of math. Wired Magazine. 2014.
34. Paul SP. Golden spirals and scalp whorls: nature's own design for rapid expansion. PLoS One. 2016;11(9):e0162026. https://doi.org/10.1371/journal.pone.0162026.
35. Baek RM, Song YT, Baek SJ, Lee JH, Im TG, Yoon BH. Effects of the recombinant human epidermal growth factor on full thickness wound of the rat skin. J Korean Soc Plast Reconstr Surg. 2003;30:201–8.

36. Park JH, Na YC, Moh JS, Lee SY, You SH. Predicting the permanent safe donor area for hair transplantation in Koreans with male pattern baldness according to the position of the parietal whorl. Arch Plast Surg. 2014;41(3):277–84. https://doi.org/10.5999/aps.2014.41.3.277.
37. Paul SP. The golden spiral flap: a new flap design that allows for closure of larger wounds under reduced tension—how studying nature's own design led to the development of a new surgical technique. Front Surg. 2016;3:63. https://doi.org/10.3389/fsurg.2016.00063.
38. Evans N, Oreffo R, Healy E, Thurner P, Man Y. Epithelial mechanobiology, skin wound healing, and the stem cell niche. J Mech Behav Biomed Mater. 2013;28:397–409.
39. Sarrazy V, Billet F, et al. Mechanisms of pathological scarring: role of myofibroblasts and current developments. Wound Repair Regen. 2011;19:s10–5.
40. Aarabi S, Bhatt KA, Shi Y, et al. Mechanical load initiates hypertrophic scar formation through decreased cellular apoptosis. FASEB J. 2007;21:3250–61.
41. Turing AM. The chemical basis of morphogenesis. Philos Trans R Soc Lond Ser B. 1952;237:37–72.
42. Sick S, Reinker S, Timmer J, Schlake T. WNT and DKK determine hair follicle spacing through a reaction-diffusion mechanism. Science. 2006;314:1447–50.
43. Paul SP. The biomechanics of behaviour. Mayo Auditorium. University of Minnesota combined Departments of Surgery Grand Rounds, 11 April 2017.
44. Ackrill JL. A New Aristotle Reader. Oxford University Press, 1988; Ch 1, p.81.

Index

© Springer International Publishing AG, part of Springer Nature 2018

185

S. P. Paul, *Biodynamic Excisional Skin Tension Lines for Cutaneous Surgery*,
https://doi.org/10.1007/978-3-319-71495-0

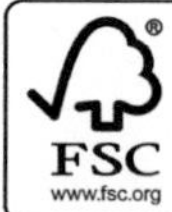